To Lori

I'm so honored to have
met you here
along the path.

THE 21-DAY YOGA BODY

→ Stay Awesome
and I'll See
you soon

♡

Mad love!!

Sadie

THE 21-DAY YOGA BODY

A Metabolic Makeover &

Life-Styling Manual to

Get You Fit, Fierce & Fabulous

in Just 3 Weeks

SADIE NARDINI

THREE RIVERS PRESS · NEW YORK

Three Rivers Press and the Tugboat design
are registered trademarks of Random House LLC.

Library of Congress Cataloging-in-Publication Data
Nardini, Sadie, 1971–
    The 21 day yoga body : a metabolic makeover and life-styling
manual to get you fit, fierce,
and fabulous in just 3 weeks / Sadie Nardini.
        pages cm
1. Yoga. I. Title.
RA781.67.N37 2013
613.7'046—dc23
                                        2013012007

ISBN 978-0-385-34706-8
eISBN 978-0-385-34707-5

Printed in the United States of America

Book design by Elizabeth Rendfleisch
Interior photographs by Francis Holland
Cover design by Jessica Sayward Bright
Cover photography by Tyler McCoy

10 9 8 7 6 5 4 3 2 1

First Edition

To my family;

all the beautiful teachers and beings

who have loved me

and allowed me

to love them in return.

There is no greater joy than this.

CONTENTS

The 21-Day Yoga Body

INTRODUCTION

What Is a Yoga Body?

Well, a yoga body is *not* an obsessive, superficial outer focus on your form only. You're not a tortilla. You're the whole enchilada, baby—and we're about to go loco on your old limiting habits.

A yoga body is freedom, freedom to be who you know you're meant to be, deep inside. It's 100-proof you, distilled to your essence on all levels, rocking your mind-bod-spirit-freakin'-entire-life to a miraculous, turbo-boosted new level. Yeah, that good.

I'm Sadie Nardini, and it's lovely to meet you.

As you'll soon find out, I've re-created my entire life to be super-naturally amazing, and I want you to do this, too. But there's something I want you to know about me—and your program—first.

This is a book about cleaning house, lighting fires, and coming home to yourself.

Outcomes you may notice over the next three weeks are: weight loss (if needed), a toned body, the ability to deal better with drama and make clear decisions about your direction, and a new eating lifestyle. But the ultimate payoff is that you're about to raise your whole vibe, heal old wounds that keep you stuck, and begin to shine so brightly that your outer reality will shift to match the shape of your spirit.

The true lifeblood coursing through this program is something as old as time—and the only thing that will work if you want to effect real changes in your life. You have to learn to *do you*.

You may not know this yet, but you are a leader. And the direction in which you lead yourself is the way you'll pull everyone and everything. Your life is only a GPS that orients to wherever you are: change your inner vibration and you'll shift your thoughts, emotions, and actions. To become the leader of mind, body, heart, and expression that you were born to be, let's get you resonating higher so that who you truly are and who you want to be become a perfect, soul-mate match—made not in heaven but right here on earth, today.

When it comes to food and exercise, the other components of a whole, hot, healthy Yoga Body, I'm not asking you to spend your life at the gym, give up what makes you happy, snack on cardboard, or aim to look freakishly perfect. I won't force you to eat kamut flakes for the rest of your life. I enjoy a good steak. I require red wine to feel complete. I believe there is a role for what you love in a healing day-to-day diet. And let's flip the script on the word *diet*, shall we? I'm sick of seeing people strip themselves of all body fat—and energy, vitality, and happiness—because they've been sold a bill of goods by pictures in a magazine.

Besides, healthy is the new skinny. The Yoga Body wants to be fit, fierce, and fabulous, inside and out. And when it comes to the "why"—your core purpose for doing anything new—think of this process less as doing something restrictive and more as doing something that gives you back everything that's really important. This is your chance to optimally fuel your vessel for greatness. After all, you have things to create, names to take, asses to kick. You'll need to be on full power to show up, every day, and create the miracles you seek.

I've designed these twenty-one days to make this major shift happen and still be easy to fit into your busy modern life. Yet all of it is rooted, like a lotus into the mud, deep in ancient yoga principles that are known to get your mojo back, fast. I'm here to translate for you, make it fun to be a badass, and invite you to break the cycle of playing small and, as my French artist friend puts it, get back to living "all zee time huge."

This is the outcome: consciously creating your best-ever Yoga Body.

WHAT DOES IT FEEL LIKE TO LIVE IN A YOGA BODY?

Like a boring ol' monk who just took a vow of silence and has nothing even resembling fun. Kidding! More like a VIP, red-hot fabulous party! Case in point: As I write this, I'm sitting on the deck of the River Café, a floating restaurant on the East River in Brooklyn. My buddy Joe Delissio, author of the *River Café Wine Primer*, set up a wine tasting for me and three of my girlfriends because, you know...we have to do *research* on your behalf for this book.

We finish with sips of a Madeira wine from 1895. Oh, baby—I just drank something that was created when Monet was still painting all his bridges and lilies. It tasted like...history.

As Patric, the maître d', and I talk about how impossible it is to rank great food, love, and wine in order, I look around myself, at my sweet friends, Joe, at the piano, out at the Brooklyn Bridge, and the slowly rolling East River, and I think to myself...This. Is. My. Life. Then I add, "Of course it is...you created it to be this way!"

Lest you think I have always lived a charmed life, as Patric would say, "au contraire, mon frère." It used to be much, much different from this.

When I was thirteen, I contracted a severe spinal cord meningitis-type illness, and it went untreated because the first diagnosis was that I had Stage IV leukemia. Yay. For several days, I thought I was going to die, until the lab realized they had put some extra zeros where they shouldn't be on my results.

The effects of the disease left me like a rag doll for two years; completely weak and unable to breathe properly, because my central nervous system was inflamed, I had five panic attacks a day on average. There was no effective treatment.

Out of desperation, my mom, Janet, aka the Black Beret—I've very rarely seen her without it on—pulled out *Richard Hittleman's Yoga: 28 Day Exercise Plan*. The lady on the cover was wearing a flesh-colored unitard. The Black Beret said, "Maybe this could help you?"

Dated fashions aside, the book saved my life. I was regularly considering ending it all and, along with it, my suffering. I had nothing to lose by hanging out in these funky poses, sometimes for hours. I couldn't even sit for long, but I sure could do the restorative poses, like lying on my back, legs up the wall, and I could breathe.

I found that the breathing techniques helped me calm my system, and I began to have fewer panic attacks. I felt a surge of hope: If I could change this one thing about myself what else was possible? And so, I began to fight.

It took me ten years to claw back up that hill into physical and mental health. But I did it, using only yoga, mindful eating, and stress-reduction techniques. I learned how to take actions that served my progress instead of retrograding me into a relapse or keeping me stuck.

Using my dedication to these same principles I'm about to teach you, I went from being on food stamps to making a high-six-figure salary, from overwhelming depression, rage, and anxiety to being just slightly irritated with certain NYC drivers some days but otherwise handling my emotional business like a Fortune 500 CEO.

Defying every prognosis, I now travel around the world doing what I love and have magical, miracle-level adventures almost every day.

If you look at me now, you may see Sadie Nardini, yogini—the handstanding, rock 'n' roll empowerment advocate with the awesome life. But make no mistake: this did not just "happen" to me.

I made this happen *for* me, every step of the way. Now I can help you make it a reality, too—if you're up for it. Because it's going to take both of us to spark the Yoga Body revolution that will start within and then ripple out and remodel every area of your life for the better.

I want nothing less than for you to become a wellness warrior: strong spine, strong body, strong mind, strong heart, strong goals, strong actions, and knowing one thing for sure—that in all matters of the mind and body, the spirit and the heart, no matter what your starting point is today, it's possible to come a loooong way, baby.

I can't wait for you to experience this brand-new, fierce you... starting now. Here's how we're going to get there.

21-DAY YOGA BODY PROGRAM

Yogis have known for centuries that to evolve in any helpful direction you must target the whole person, not merely one part, like just diet or only exercise. Without systemic transformation, the shift feels empty and incomplete, like when you try to high-five someone and miss.

Here, we address the whole you. To do this most effectively, we'll follow the road map of Patanjali (let's just call him "Pat")—an ancient yoga philosopher who wrote the Yoga Sutras, a guide to centered living.

In Sanskrit, Pat described three major steps to transformation, collectively known as Kriya Yoga, or the yoga of rocking your world in any and every way. The three steps are

Tapas (tuh-pas): *Presence, New Energy.* Train your senses to get with the program in the midst of challenge. Become high-quality present. Make space. Unlock and contain energy. Ignite your life force to burn away obstacles to center.

Svadhyaya (svahd-hyai-yah): *Inner Inquiry, Truth, Center.* Go inside. Get authentic. Access your creative source. Discover your core truths, or *satya* (suht-ya). Self-nourish and take counsel from your inner teacher.

Ishvara Pranidhana (ish-vahr-ah prahnee-dhan-ah): *Aligned Action, Surrender.* Offer your truth to the world. Take action for its own sake and trust that when you represent your truth in any situation the best possible outcome for all participants is assured.

These three guideposts to converting your frustrations into positive energetic currency are found everywhere. For example, consider this part of the Serenity Prayer by Reinhold Niebuhr:

God, grant me the serenity
to accept the things I cannot change, [Ishvara Pranidhana]
The courage to change the things I can, [Tapas]
And wisdom to know the difference. [Svadhyaya]

When it comes to becoming your truth, there are many doorways in, and there is no separation between what you practice in one aspect of your life and all the rest. I'm here to transmute these classical concepts into steps you can take, today, to do what you came here to do: create the freedom to love your life and be yourself so fully that you can leave this world with a crazy-big grin on your face and no regrets.

YOUR RESULTS AND HOW TO GET THERE

Each week, you'll focus on one of the three steps. I've renamed them from the Sanskrit terms so that you don't have to speak in tongues (unless you like that sort of thing).

WEEK ONE: Foundation

WEEK TWO: Core

WEEK THREE: Expression

What you'll do:
- A brand-new, engaging, and fun yoga practice, designed by me, an anatomy geek, to give you the most safety, strength, stretch, and balance results from the time you spend on the mat.

- Daily inspiration about how to approach your challenges and relationships—and rock them.

- A daily meal plan that gives you a new, creative relationship with food and tons of information on how to eat fresh, whole, and fantastically well for a lifetime.

- Action steps to make all these great ideas a reality in your day-to-day life.

What you'll get:
- Increased core strength inside and out: a strong spine literally and figuratively, higher self-esteem, a renewed fierceness of spirit, and the ability to know yourself more deeply and trust what you hear.

∴ Weight loss, probably. Increased physical fitness for sure. Many participants lose ten to fifteen pounds of pure fat and add toned lean muscle mass, that elusive magic metabolism combination.

Important Tips to Help Get the Most Out of Your 21-Day Program

Hell yes you *can* fit this program into your busy life. You already grocery shop, think, eat, make meals, and do stuff all day long anyway. We are just re-organizing and refocusing your same actions in a different way to get you the results you want. Also, you were born to be real, not perfect, so do what you can. Even small changes will make a big difference.

Here's how to organize yourself each day and reallocate your energy to get the most out of the program.

1. Every morning, take a look at the daily theme and action steps. Reflect on them for a few minutes. Think about how you'll fit the adventure ideas in today.

2. Do your yoga whenever you can, but do it. The minimum is 30 minutes a day—I'd love for you to do more. The more time you invest in your yoga practice, ideally up to 1 hour 5 to 6 times a week, the more mind/body returns you will get. I find that doing yoga in the a.m. is best, because then it's out of the way. If you wait till you're knackered from a busy day, it'll be a crapshoot.

3. Eat regular meals and snacks. I know we all skip them sometimes—but do your best to plan ahead and eat consistently to keep your metabolism stoked, especially for these 21 days.

4. Hydrate well. It makes all systems go more efficiently and keeps you energized and detoxifying 24/7.

5. Eat dinner early enough—two hours before bed, at least, so that you digest before you go to sleep.

6. Preparation is key. Look at the next day the night before. Do your food prep; if you work, prepare your lunch to take to work the evening before, rather than scrambling in the morning.

7. Get to bed early. I know it's hard, but do it anyway. It makes all the difference. Use my meditations and themes to deflect drama and get to sleep faster.

8. Try to meditate at least 10 minutes in the morning. The turbo-charged clarity, refreshed mind, and reduced stress (hormones) all day long is worth one snooze button push.

Every day of the program includes a *Daily Inspiration* and a *Yoga Body Meal Plan*. Read the Daily Inspiration in the morning, before you meditate, and reflect on it then and during the day. The Yoga Body Meal Plan is a whole new way of being with food and will rev up your metabolism so it will work for you, not against you. Because guess what? Dieting bites the big one, *and* it doesn't work.

This program gets you back to the earth, to organic, simple eating that your body understands. I lost forty pounds switching my diet to this non-diet, which tastes way better yet supports, not sabotages, my fitness efforts—and I'll offer you all of my secrets: basic recipes that you can customize, common diet pitfalls to avoid, quick meals to throw together, and easy food and beverage ideas from my personal stash.

Believe me, I've tried it all to get my body to look hot and be healthy at the same time. For six years—*years*—I used to eat nothing but vegetables and tried to keep my calories low so that I'd stay thin enough to go out in public wearing yoga tights for a living. I felt tired, cranky, and sick. I ate 1,200 calories a day, not enough to fuel my brain or organs. But I was a size 4.

I hooked up with two amazing nutritionists—Jenn Pike, RHN, and Dr. Kristen Bentson—who supported me to drop my depleting diet and make the switch to an energy-fueling food lifestyle. The process of moving back into a life-affirming meal plan, still having fun and also eating enough to power my activity level, forms the basis of what I'll share with you in this program.

Now I eat about 2,000 calories a day, a ton of healing foods—and I'm a lean, toned size 6 who feels she can take on the world. Size doesn't matter, ladies; this is mine, but you'll get to your best number for your frame when you eat enough and enough quality to reach all your fitness goals.

These days, when people meet me and find out that I'm a yoga and ultimate wellness expert, they are about as surprised at that (most yoga teachers don't have a Mohawk and ride around on a boy's BMX bike, apparently) as they are to find that I'm a wine geek and love a good free-range steak once a week. OK . . . twice.

Get ready to throw out those pasty, fat-free cookies, and throw a wine and cheese party instead. A truly balanced diet can look much different from what we may have been taught. I'm not selling you a remove-this, restrict-that *diet*—one that's dull as dust and tastes about as good. When it comes to helping your body help itself to look strong and feel alive rather than exhausted, going to extremes in any way is not the answer. I don't like saying "no" forever to things I enjoy just to have a nice ass. I believe that your eating plan should give you a head-swiveling outer form but also make you feel energized and inspired inside.

Yay! I can't wait for you to experience how good it feels to eat and drink the New Healthy way.

Core Strength Vinyasa Yoga

I've spent the last two decades studying with some of the best yoga and anatomy experts there are, formulating a style—Core Strength Vinyasa Yoga—that contains the most cutting-edge alignment and holistic anatomy instructions, which you won't find anywhere else.

Whatever type of yoga you do now, you can benefit from this style, which will both complement and enhance your current style.

Just know that if you want to be strong, be safe, and get more benefits, you'll have to move differently than you may have been previously taught in old-school trainings. This is your new school yoga evolution!

Every day you'll get a new, creative mini-flow to add to your daily Yoga Body Warm-Up, Core Sun Salutation, and Cooldown to keep you building lean muscle, burning fat, and gaining more flexibility.

Daily Action Adventures

What will make the difference between this being the most body-mind-life-rocking book you ever bought and just another block of paper that sits on your shelf making your dinner guests think you're all spiritual and stuff? Busting a move.

You can't sit on your keister and expect things to change. You have to *do* something differently, in the direction of your goals.

So when you read my action step for the day, or when it comes to actually buying and making great meals for yourself or getting your asana up off the couch and onto that mat, it's up to you to muster the drive to make a shift.

I worked hard to make the Action Adventures both fun and super-duper easy for you; however, they are each included on purpose—to flick your Bic in a deep way and light up the foundational core strength that is built only when you take self-empowering actions.

For example, you're not just making a bath cocktail sachet and tossing it in the tub. You're making a direct statement to your Self that you are worth loving. Take enough of these new actions and you'll transform into a habitually outrageous, consistently courageous rock star. The necklace of your life is built one bead at a time, right here and now.

YOGA BODY BASICS

How Your Meal Plan Will Work Best

FOOD & DRINK

Before you move, on or off the yoga mat, it's important to first fuel yourself properly to get the best results. The Meal templates that follow give you the power to keep creating healthy meals as a lifestyle for a lifetime. I want you to learn through creative repetition and recipes-with-room how to make every meal work for you.

Also, you can mix and match any recipe within the week for which you've purchased the groceries from the Pantry Lists; so if you feel like the smoothie from Day 3 for lunch on Day 6, be my guest.

As long as you're using fresh, quality ingredients and not veering wildly from the basic recipe (adding a cup of sugar and a bag of chocolate chips to the quinoa protein bars, for example, or eating from the Avoid List) you're good.

If you're eating out, try to approximate the types and sizes of meals on this program: fresh, whole foods; not a lot of sauces; and a mix of protein, complex carbs, and healthy fats. The lists of food types that follow will give you some options.

You can always make more of any dish and take it to work the next day, too.

Here are the food and yoga guidelines you'll use every day of the program.

A Word on Weight Loss

This is not a calorie-restricted, weight loss program. It's sensitivity training for your palate, your body, and your health.

Make sure to check out www.21DayYogaBody .com for tons of additional fresh, fierce, and fabulous recipes.

When you eat a whole-food diet and eat just until you're satisfied, not stuffed, you are not likely to gain—or sustain—unhealthy amounts of weight. Many people tell me they lose excess weight naturally on this program, although losing weight just to be skinny is never my aim. It's my intention to make you fit, strong, energetic, and "belly-happy" at your body's natural set point—not imbalanced on either side of the scale.

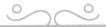

Definition of Food Types

PROTEIN: lean meats, beans, lentils, quinoa (a high-protein seed), organic tofu, seitan, tempeh, nuts, and nut butter (cashew, almond, peanut, sunflower)

WHOLE-FOOD GRAINS: any whole rice (brown, red, black), quinoa (technically, a seed), amaranth, Kamut, barley, buckwheat, millet, rolled oats, oat groats, spelt, wheat berries, and teff

SALAD GREENS: spinach, arugula, romaine lettuce, red leaf lettuce, Bibb lettuce, watercress, kale, mixed wild greens

COOKING GREENS: spinach, arugula, kale, collard, Swiss chard, dandelion, cabbage, beet greens, escarole

HEALTHY FATS FOR COOKING: extra-virgin olive oil, canola oil, extra-virgin coconut oil, flaxseed oil, avocado oil, organic butter

HEALTHY FATS: all the fats just listed, plus nut oils (like hazelnut or pumpkin seed), fish oil, actual avocado, all nuts, seeds (like pumpkin or sunflower), and limited amounts of eggs and aged or organic cheese

ALTERNATIVE MILKS: coconut, almond, oat, hemp, rice, soy; if you drink animal milk, ensure that it's growth-hormone-free and preferably organic

FRUIT: fresh or dried, unsulfured, unsweetened fruit of any variety

DAIRY: organic cheese, fresh or aged (limited amounts) and yogurt. If you're lactose intolerant, goat's milk or aged cheeses are often easier to digest

General Meal Guidelines

Most meals, drinks, or snacks optimally should include:

- protein
- whole-food, complex carbohydrate (vegetables, fruit, beans/legumes, whole grains)
- healthy fat
- fun, inspiring stuff, such as a sprinkle of cheese or the aforementioned chocolate chips

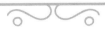

Menu Basics: Creating Your Meals & Drinks

These are suggested ways to compose different drinks or dishes; a road map of what you might put in each type of meal as you move through the 21 days.

FRESH JUICES: I didn't mention many of these, since we're trying not to break your bank. But if you can get a juicer or go to a local juice bar, I highly recommend it. You can also throw these ingredients into a blender; you'll get a more smoothie-like texture, or you can strain the mixture. Fresh fruit and vegetable juice is an amazing meal or snack substitute to give your body the enzymes and nutrients it needs to heal and cleanse. If you juice, here are some of my favorites blends.

> **EYE GLASS** (great for vision): beet, carrot, orange, mint
>
> **GREEN GODDESS** (a detox-o-rama): cucumber, spinach, kale, celery, lemon, apple
>
> **PURPLE PASSION:** blackberries, raspberries, beet, blueberry, apple
>
> **ORANGE YOU HEALTHY:** pineapple, mango, orange, a splash of lemon
>
> **GREEN MARIA:** green or red tomatoes, spinach, cilantro, black pepper or cayenne, a pinch of sea salt, lime; blend this one until pureed

It's hard to say how much you need, since fruits and veggies vary in size. Experiment until you hit the recipe that works for you, but, in general, choose from

- 4 cups leafy greens
- 1 to 2 medium-size pieces each of fruit or water-based veggies, like mango or cucumber
- a 1-inch cube of peeled fresh ginger (optional)
- pinch of spice: cinnamon, cayenne, salt, pepper
- half to a whole lemon or lime, squeezed

If you have a juicer (suggested), feed all veggie and fruit ingredients through it as usual, including the ginger. Add any lemon, spices, or seasonings at the end.

If you're using a blender, peel any veggies or fruits that require it, like mangoes, oranges, and the like. Remove any hard pits. Chop everything into rough

A Note About Fresh Juices: As full of goodness as fruit and sweeter veggie juices are, they can still cause a blast of blood sugar and insulin into the system. Drink them in moderation, or, optimally, balanced with fats, fiber, and protein.

pieces. Put all the ingredients into the blender, and alternate blending on Low and High until pureed.

Pour the puree into a large microstrainer set over a bowl. Stir the puree periodically for a few minutes until juice collects in the bowl. You can also pour the mix into cheesecloth or a thin towel over a bowl, fold the towel edges over the mix, and squeeze the juice into the bowl. Pour into a glass over ice and drink up.

SMOOTHIE BASICS

Your goal is to see how many balanced nutrients and how much vitality you can fit into one glass, fast.

2 cups fresh or frozen fruit

ice, if not using frozen fruit

1 cup milk or alternative

½ cup filtered water or to desired consistency (I also recommend coconut water for added electrolytes)

1 teaspoon honey or agave nectar (optional)

1 tablespoon flax oil, if not including nuts

1 to 2 cups spinach leaves or de-stemmed kale

protein of choice (either 1 scoop of Vega One or other protein powder supplement, 1 tablespoon nuts or nut butter, 1 cup yogurt, or 1 cup silken organic tofu)

1 capsule probiotics and/or digestive enzymes (break capsule and shake into smoothie)

Place frozen fruit or fresh fruit and ice into the blender first. Add all liquids and then the rest of your ingredients.

Blend on High for 30 seconds and then Low for 30 seconds, alternating until the desired consistency is reached. Pour into a tall glass and serve.

FRICKTTATA BASICS

Serves 4, or 1 with leftovers

Otherwise known as a frittata, this one's so frickin' fast I had to rename it. You'll get a whole lot of nutrition in not a lot of time, including an optimal balance of fats and protein from eating the whole egg, not only the white. You can mix and match the ingredients you like, and if you don't have fresh herbs, use a dash of dried. Save some and eat it cold or reheat in an olive-oiled pan on medium heat for a quick meal or snack.

8 organic eggs

1/2 cup grated or crumbled cheese

3 large fresh basil leaves, minced

3 large fresh sage leaves, minced

1 teaspoon minced fresh rosemary

1/4 teaspoon sea salt

1/8 teaspoon freshly ground black pepper

3 tablespoons extra-virgin olive oil

2 cups finely sliced or chopped mixed veggies of choice (try red bell pepper, red onion, green onion, spinach, asparagus tips, zucchini, sundried tomatoes)

2 cloves garlic, minced (optional)

1 tablespoon salsa, sour cream, or splash of hot sauce (optional)

Preheat the oven to 400°F.

In a medium bowl, mix together eggs, cheese, herbs, and salt and pepper. In a medium ovenproof saucepan, heat oil on medium-high heat. Add veggies and garlic; and sauté until soft, about 6 minutes. Reduce heat to low.

Pour in egg mixture, and stir once to mix. Cook until frittata begins to set, about 2 minutes. Do not further scramble or stir. Place in oven; bake until just set, 7 to 9 minutes.

Slide the frittata onto a platter. Cut into wedges and serve at any temperature with desired accompaniments. Keep the rest in your fridge, well-wrapped, for up to 3 days.

SALAD BASICS

A staple of any healthy diet, salads are invigoration in a bowl. Mix and match a variety of ingredients, and change them up each week to get the maximum benefits.

2 to 4 cups organic salad greens

2 cups fresh chopped veggies of choice

1/2 cup fresh or dried fruit

1/4 cup nuts

1/4 cup organic cheese

1/2 cup dressing of your choice (see recipes that follow)

pinch fresh cracked black pepper, or to taste

Place all ingredients except dressing and pepper in a medium bowl. Toss lightly to mix.

Serve on a separate plate or bowl, and drizzle with the dressing here, not in the mixing bowl. Add pepper to taste. Nondressed leftovers (dressing wilts the lettuce) will keep longer in the fridge.

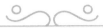

SALAD DRESSING BASICS

Any dressing that has the following elements will rock:

- ❖ a base of healthy oil
- ❖ complementary ingredients added to taste, such as pureed fruit, mustard, vinegar, yogurt, cheese (though not in the same recipe, yuck!)
- ❖ herbs and seasonings to taste: garlic, pepper, sea salt, rosemary, and the like

---

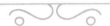

Here are five of my go-to dressings.

CARROT-MISO-GINGER DRESSING

This miso-based, nutrition-and-digestive-enzyme-packed dressing can be used over salads, rice, and veggie dishes, and even as a sandwich spread. It's so good, I'd take a bath in it if I could.

4 tablespoons rice vinegar

4 tablespoons water

3 tablespoons white miso paste

1 carrot, chopped into medium pieces

1 teaspoon peeled, chopped fresh ginger

1 teaspoon chopped garlic

Place all ingredients in a blender. Blend on High for 20 seconds and then Low for 20 more seconds, or until the desired consistency is reached.

Pour into a serving container. Store any extra in the fridge in a sealed container. Keeps for a few days.

BADASS BALSAMIC VINAIGRETTE

This was the first dressing I learned to make, and I still use it constantly.

½ cup extra-virgin olive oil

½ cup balsamic vinegar

1 teaspoon mustard

1 clove garlic, crushed

Sea salt and freshly ground black pepper to taste

Optional: 1 teaspoon honey or 1 teaspoon minced fresh rosemary or 1 teaspoon minced scallions and 2 teaspoons grated Parmesan cheese

Whisk together all the ingredients in a measuring cup or small bowl. Or put all the ingredients into an almost empty mustard jar and shake vigorously. Store leftover dressing in a sealed container in the fridge. Keeps for up to a week.

CREAMY GARLIC DRESSING

This creamy delight also serves as a dip for raw veggies or can be poured over any skillet salad or quinoa/rice bowl dish. Plus, it's vegan, so it's perfect for those who are dairy- and egg-free or lactose intolerant.

1/3 cup cashews

2 cups filtered water

juice of half a lemon

1 tablespoon wheat-free tamari or
    soy sauce

1 tablespoon minced fresh dill or parsley
    (optional)

2 cloves garlic, minced

Place the cashews in small bowl. Pour the filtered water over them to just cover. Set a kitchen towel over the bowl, and let the cashews soak for at least as long as it takes you to prep the other ingredients or overnight in the fridge.

Blend all of the ingredients on Pulse for 30 seconds or until smooth. Store the dressing in a sealed container in the fridge. Keeps for up to a week.

ROCKIN' RASPBERRY VINAIGRETTE

This tangy, fruity dressing is a lovely addition to your salads, especially ones that contain nuts.

1/4 cup extra-virgin olive oil

1/4 cup apple cider vinegar

1/4 cup organic apple juice or cider

2 tablespoons honey

3/4 cup raspberries (fresh or frozen)

Put all liquid ingredients into a blender, and puree until smooth.

Add the raspberries last, and blend on Low to desired consistency. Store leftover dressing in a sealed container in the fridge. Keeps for up to a week.

5-MINUTE SHAKE 'N' SERVE LIGHT VINAIGRETTE

This sweet-and-savory dressing contains heart-healthy olive oil, and the Dijon binds it perfectly for a smooth, tangy dressing.

½ cup red wine vinegar	1 teaspoon Dijon mustard
1½ cups olive oil	½ clove garlic, crushed
½ teaspoon sea salt	½ teaspoon fresh rosemary, minced
½ teaspoon honey	¼ cup grated Parmesan cheese
¼ teaspoon black pepper	

Combine all ingredients in a Mason or other glass jar with a screw-on lid. Immediately before serving, tighten lid and shake vigorously until entirely mixed. Keeps for 4 days in the fridge.

GRAINS BASICS

SADIE'S RICE COOKER CASSEROLE *OR* SKILLET SALAD

I designed the following two dishes to give you the maximum nutrition in the minimum amount of cooking time. It's fun to play with the ingredients, so mix and match as you wish to create your own signature favorites.

I love my rice cooker, and I suggest you get one, because it multitasks so many meals, but you can do these on your stove, as well.

The Beautiful Body Bowl (uses a rice cooker)

½ cup quinoa or other grain	2 to 4 cups sliced, assorted veggies and protein
1¼ cups water	sea salt, pepper, or other seasoning to taste
dash olive oil	

Add the grain, water, salt, and oil to the bottom of the rice cooker and cook according to directions.

After 5 to 10 minutes, add the protein to the bottom of the steamer tray, and then cover with veggies and set on top of the grain. Cover and let steamer cook until ready.

When done, place some grain in a bowl, cover with the veggies and protein, and add any additional salt, pepper, or seasoning (for example, balsamic vinegar, hot sauce, dressing, olive oil, lemon). Stir together and enjoy.

Skillet Salad (If you don't have a rice cooker, use a pan!)

1 cup grain of choice (I use wild or brown rice or quinoa)

filtered water according to package directions

pinch of sea salt

3 teaspoons olive oil

2 cups mixed, chopped fruit, veggies, or nuts of choice (peas, raisins, dried cranberries, zucchini, mushrooms, onions, edamame beans, garlic, carrots, cashews, hazelnuts, almonds, walnuts, and pine nuts all work well)

8 ounces protein of choice, sliced (I often use chicken sausage, tofu, or steak, or fry one egg in the middle of the skillet)

2 cups cooking greens (optional)

seasonings of choice (hot sauce, balsamic vinegar, any leftover salad dressing, sea salt, and pepper) to taste

In your pot, mix together your grain, water, and sea salt. Cook the grain according to the package directions.

In a sauté pan over medium-high, heat the olive oil until a piece of garlic thrown in sizzles. Add any garlic, onions next, and sauté until slightly brown. Add any other veggies, nuts, protein. Stir in any seasoning.

Sauté until protein browns and veggies are slightly soft. Add any greens on top, remove from heat, and cover for 1 to 2 minutes or until greens wilt.

When the grain is cooked, place the desired amount into a bowl. Stir it together with some of the same seasoning that you used for the skillet mix.

Place desired amount of skillet mix on top of the grain or mix everything together. Garnish with more seasoning, and serve.

I always make a little more than I need. You can store the extras in the fridge for up to 3 days, so you'll have something ready-made when you're busy (and hungry).

DETOX-TAIL BEVERAGES BASICS

When you want to flush-out your system, have a Detox-tail. This is a cocktail that has detox properties. It should include

⅓ cup fresh or frozen fruit

liquid of choice (choose 2 that
    go together, 4 ounces each)
    filtered water, fizzy water
    (seltzer, soda water, sparkling
    water), tea (herbal, black,
    green), fresh fruit or veggie
    juice

1 teaspoon honey or agave nectar
    (optional)

Put the fruit in a tall 8- to 12-ounce cocktail glass. If fruit is frozen, no ice is needed; otherwise, add ice to fill half of the glass.

Add any juice or other liquid next to fill glass three-quarters of the way. Finish with seltzer water or milk (if appropriate), any sweetener, and stir to mix. Garnish with lemon or lime if desired and a happy flair—a little paper umbrella usually works. If you want to make your Detox-tail into a proper cocktail, add 1 ounce of vodka, sake, tequila, or any other clear, preferably organic, liquor. The clearer, the cleaner.

A note on adding sweeteners

Agave nectar, honey, raw sugar, and maple syrup are simple carbs, but they come from more natural sources than manufactured fake sugars. In my opinion, unless you can't eat sugars for some reason, even white table sugar is better for your body than aspartame, Splenda, or other sugar substitutes—at least your body recognizes it as real food. This is why I suggest eating the real deal but pairing it with something that contains fiber and protein, like putting it over quinoa or sprinkling some raw sugar into your protein-added coconut milk chai latte.

So please, throw away the fake sugars. I'd rather see you eat a little real food sweetener, or none at all, than chemically degrade your health. That's drama we can all avoid.

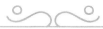

DESSERT BASICS

Even your Yoga Body desserts should include
- protein and whole carbohydrates
- healthy forms of fats and sweeteners (avocados and dark chocolate or cocoa powder instead of processed milk and chocolate)
- no guilt—only enjoying to the max

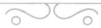

AVOID LIST

You can have any of these you want, I'm not here to stop you, but eat enough of these foods and your body and health will begin to reflect them in weight gain, fatigue, and inflammation. So maybe you don't want them so much anymore. Hence, I invite you to avoid the following as much as you can:

- fake sugars, such as sucralose and aspartame; eat real food sweeteners (raw sugar, honey, agave nectar, whole fruit) or none at all

- diet soda and most chewing gum

- regular soda, all drinks containing high-fructose corn syrup and other over-processed sugars (this includes many sports drinks and bottled juices)

- anything that you don't recognize as nature-made food or that lasts for months on the shelf (this should take care of most other unhealthy fats, chemicals, and ingredients I could mention . . . but probably can't spell; as unprocessed as possible is always best)

- nonorganic animal milk or animal milk with growth hormones and products made with it

- anything that your stomach and body tells you it doesn't like through headaches, bloating, pain, nausea, cramping, or digestive issues

PREPARE YOURSELF AND YOUR PANTRY

The following lists are the foods you'll need to rock the 21 days. Prepping your pantry is your first Action Adventure. Remember, this is not a shopping list; it is a self-healing and loving mission . . . if you choose to accept it.

I don't always say this in the recipes, but when you shop for any item, choose organic whenever possible. When you eat high-quality food, your body will get the nutrients it needs, and you will not be as hungry or crave as much food as when you eat nutritionally substandard items. Plus, potentially avoiding diet-related illness later is well worth a few extra dollars now.

Before you shop, take a look at your Yoga Body Recipes. If you aren't going to make some of the meals, don't like certain ingredients, or don't eat meat, for example, then cross those items off the list or substitute other things within the program that you like.

If you don't have a large refrigerator or freezer, you'll want to shop for some of the perishable items once or twice a week. Fish is best bought the day you're going to cook it.

This list is only for you, with the exception of a few family meals for two to four people. Get more if you'll be cooking for others.

Wine 'n' Dine

Maybe it's my Italian heritage or just a personal fascination, but nevertheless, I'm asking you to geek out on wine with me—in moderation.

A glass of wine here and there with your meals can be part of a healthy diet and, in fact, add to it. Wine is full of antioxidants and fat-dissolving compounds in addition to good cheer! Of course, if you don't drink wine, we have plenty of other fun beverages for you to try.

Opening your mind and palate to learning more about the grape is just another way to explore your trust, creativity, and individuality and to amp up the experience of your life from merely pleasant to passionate.

DRY GOODS (FOR ALL 3 WEEKS):

Canned Goods:
1 (8-ounce) can refried beans
2 (8-ounce) cans organic cannellini beans
2 (8-ounce) cans organic black beans
4 (8-ounce) cans organic chickpeas
1 (8-ounce) can organic green beans
1 (8-ounce) can organic whole-kernel corn
1 (14.7-ounce) can organic chili

Spices:
1 (4.7-ounce) jar salt
1 (2.3-ounce) jar black pepper
1 (2.3-ounce) jar red pepper flakes
1 (2.9-ounce) jar paprika
1 (1.7-ounce) jar cayenne pepper
1 (4-ounce) bottle organic vanilla extract
1 (2.4-ounce) jar cinnamon

Grains:
1 (14-ounce) bag flaxseeds
2 (12-ounce) boxes quinoa
quarter-pound chia seeds
1 (32-ounce) bag gluten-free rolled oats
1 (2-pound) bag brown rice
1 (16-ounce) box gluten-free spaghetti noodles
1 (32-ounce) bag buckwheat flour
1 (12-ounce) package gluten-free hamburger
    buns

Oils:
1 (16-ounce) bottle canola oil
1 (25.4-ounce) bottle extra-virgin olive oil
1 (16-ounce) bottle extra-virgin coconut oil
1 (16-ounce) bottle flaxseed oil

Condiments:
1 (23.5-ounce) bottle agave nectar
1 (8-ounce) bottle honey
1 (8-ounce) bottle maple syrup
1 (8-ounce) bottle red wine vinegar
1 (10-ounce) bottle soy sauce or wheat-free
    tamari
1 (12.7-ounce) bottle dark sesame oil

1 (17-ounce) bottle balsamic vinegar
1 (12-ounce) jar nut butter
1 (8-ounce) jar Dijon mustard
1 (12-ounce) bottle organic chocolate syrup
1 (2.3-ounce) jar nutmeg
1 (24-ounce) jar canola mayonnaise

Nuts:
1 (17-ounce) package of Marcona almonds
½ pound pepitas
1 pound raw almonds or nuts of choice
1 (8-ounce) bag cashews

Dried Fruit:
1 (16-ounce) bag dried fruit of choice (dates,
    cherries, raisins, cranberries)

Add Ins:
1 (30.8-ounce) container protein powder or
    Vega One Vanilla Chai mix
1 (8-ounce) bag shredded coconut
1 (3-ounce) jar pimentos
1 (3.5-ounce) jar capers
1 (8-ounce) jar Kalamata olives
1 (16-ounce) container cocoa powder
1 (1.7-ounce) bag wakame (sea vegetable) or
    dried wakame

Drinks:
1 box tea (with 16 tea bags each of green tea,
    berry tea, matcha tea, and chai tea)
2 (2-liter) bottles seltzer water
1 liter coconut water

Other:
1 (6-ounce) container cornstarch, tapioca, or
    arrowroot starch
1 (12.1-ounce) tube organic white miso
1 (3.2-ounce) chocolate bar with 70% cacao
    or higher
1 (14-ounce) bag corn tortillas
1 (16-ounce) bag brown sugar
1 (32-ounce) carton chicken stock or
    vegetable broth
1 (8-ounce) container baking soda

Optional:

probiotics, digestive enzymes in capsule or
    liquid form
1 cup macadamia nuts
1.7-ounce container Herbes de Provence
1 (5-ounce) bottle hot sauce
1 (16-ounce) container vanilla protein powder
    (hemp if you can get it)
1 (8-ounce) bag poppy seeds
1 (16-ounce) bag sesame seeds
1 (7-ounce) can jalapeño slices
1 (7.5-ounce) jar cornichon pickles

WEEK 1
Meat & Meat Alternatives:
12 to 16 ounces mahimahi
1 (6-ounce) fillet mahimahi
6 ounces protein of choice
1 pack organic turkey or veggie bacon

Dairy and Dairy Alternatives:
½ gallon carton almond milk or coconut milk
1 (35.3-ounce) tub Greek yogurt
5- to 7-ounce block of cheese

Fruits & Veggies:
5 lemons
3 limes
1 small container cherry tomatoes
9 ripe tomatoes
1 small bunch celery
1 bag baby carrots
2 jalapeño peppers
½ cup green peas
1 bunch kale
4 ripe avocados
2 cucumbers
1 orange/red bell pepper
1 yellow onion
2 red onions
1 small bunch scallions
1 zucchini
2 bananas

2 oranges
6 apples
2 cups ripe seedless watermelon
2 mangoes
1 bunch each fresh dill, cilantro, rosemary,
    basil, sage (or get small spice jars of dried)
1 head garlic
1 ginger root
2 bags spinach
1 bag arugula

Fridge:
half-gallon carton orange juice
1 dozen eggs

Freezer:
½ gallon dairy-free ice cream
1 (10-ounce) bag frozen peaches
3 (10-ounce) bags frozen berries

WEEK 2
Meat & Meat Alternatives:
4 (6-ounce) salmon fillets
2 (6-ounce) whitefish fillets
1 (6-ounce) fish fillet or other protein

Dairy and Dairy Alternatives:
1 (35.3-ounce) tub Greek yogurt
5- to 7-ounce block of cheese
½ gallon carton milk or alternative

Fruits & Veggies:
1 bag arugula
1 bag spinach
1 head garlic
1 cup cubed papaya or mango
1 Ruby Red grapefruit
1 banana
1 tangerine or citrus fruit of your choice
1 red onion
1 bag edamame
1 portobello mushroom
1 red pepper
1 yellow pepper

1 head red cabbage
2 medium zucchini
1 bunch asparagus
1 large carrot
1 cucumber
1 (12-ounce) container cherry tomatoes
2 green apples
1 (12-ounce) container berries
1 head cauliflower
5 lemons
3 limes
1 avocado
1 green apple
1 papaya

Fridge:
1 dozen eggs

Freezer:
2 (10-ounce) bags frozen mango
1 (10-ounce) bag frozen berries
1 (10-ounce) bag frozen pineapple

WEEK 3
Meat & Meat Alternatives:
6 ounces Maine lobster meat (two tails)
2 burger patties (try pre-made organic
    ground beef, lamb, buffalo, turkey, or
    ostrich)
2 to 3 cups rotisserie chicken meat
2 (4- to 6-ounce) fish fillets

Dairy and Dairy Alternatives:
1/2 gallon coconut or almond milk
5- to 7-ounce block cheese of choice (try
    Parmesan)
1 (35.3-ounce) tub Greek yogurt

Fruits & Veggies:
1 bag spinach
1 bag arugula
2 bunches kale
1 medium-size potato
4 scallions

1 green or red apple
4 pears
4 cups dates
1 peach
1 (12-ounce) container blackberries
1 bunch fresh oregano
1 bunch seedless green or red grapes
1 red bell pepper
3 avocados
2 red onions
4 yellow onions
1 white onion
5 carrots
1 bunch celery
6 tomatoes
5 green tomatoes
1 bunch shallots
1 small bunch fresh oregano
1 head garlic
4 cups whole green beans
1 ear corn
1 mango
2 lemons
2 limes
2 ounces shredded red cabbage
1 jalapeño
5 ancho chiles (dried poblano pepper)
1 bunch bananas
1 cucumber

Fridge:
1 dozen eggs

Freezer:
6 ounces organic fresh or frozen shrimp
1 (12-ounce) bag frozen dark cherries or
    berries
1 (16-ounce) bag frozen peaches

YOGA BASICS

For your most effective
yoga practice, you'll
need some things (see
my favorite props at
www.21DayYogaBody
.com):

- a sticky yoga mat with
  a good, grippy surface
- a yoga block or two
- bare feet (you want
  the grounding and foot
  health that comes from
  working as nature
  intended: no socks, no
  shoes)
- an outfit that lets you
  move yet is formfitting

YOGA BODY 101

You're about to embark on a mega-effective, new evolution of yoga. And I want you to know exactly why. Many exercise movements these days, yoga included, are not as effective as they could be, and some of them are downright dangerous. That's because we overuse parts and pieces of our outer body, and neglect the deeper core muscle body. What do I mean by this?

Core strength is widely misunderstood. It's not just your abs. In fact, we now know that your muscles are each covered by Spidey-suit-like connective tissue called fascia (fash-uh). This stuff is awesome. It connects some muscles to others through the joints, in lines or meridians, from feet to head. This is important to know when you practice yoga, because some meridians, like the outermost-front and back-body ones (basically anything you can feel as you run your hands over your body), should not be overused for support in yoga poses.

Powering through your practice—or any movement—by gripping into more obvious outer-body meridians (think: quads, glutes, lower back, chest, shoulders) can cause your spine and joints to strain, make inflammation or injury more likely, and create more tension instead of real strength.

There is one meridian that isn't often talked about, but it's your deepest source of whole-body core strength. I call it the Core Strength Muscle Meridian, also called the Core Strength Meridian or Core

Body, interchangeably; it is the line of muscles closer to your bones, pelvis, and spine, and it's built to hold you in alignment and move you more safely, strongly, and fluidly.

To access your Core Body, you must first relax your outer muscles, move closer to the floor by bending your arms and legs, and activate your Core Strength Muscle Meridian from the ground up and the inside out. Only then do you firm your outer body around this inner yoga pose—to support your core strength, not to take over for it.

Don't worry if you don't understand exactly what I mean while you're reading this; as you move through the 21 days of the program, you will experience it for yourself. Just follow my instructions, move a little differently than you may be used to in your poses, and you'll unlock a whole world of new results, like increased muscle tone, less joint compression, greater power and lightness in each posture, and an increase in detoxification and digestion that will help you feel clean and clear, even as you transform from the inside out.

When you wave smoothly through my three steps to activate the Core Body—from Foundation (whatever's on the floor) to Core (pelvis and low back spine) up the spine or the rest of the pose into Expression—you'll get the best benefits possible from your time spent on the mat.

These are the main Core Strength Muscle Meridian points we seek to activate, in the following order:

Things to Remember on Your Mat

Breathe slowly and deeply through your nose using the Belly Bonfire Breath (see page 30) in all poses until you rest at the end.

If any move is too hard, take it down a notch: put a knee down, stand up higher, don't go so far into the movement, or rest in Child's Pose whenever you need to.

The point is not to be able to do every pose like a pro today. Be where you are, respect your boundaries, and don't push, but press your edge. This is how you'll chip away at the poses and gain healthy strength and flexibility over time.

The goal is to work out without burning out. Many fitness trends today tend toward super-agro, but this is not the only way to get results. Even a strong yoga workout should center you, not agitate your system or trigger you into fight or flight. This can trip your stress hormones and cause weight gain and other illnesses. Stay active but balanced and breathing.

You're not just doing a body movement. Each of these poses is a chance to practice putting the theme of the day into your actual experience. Keep it in mind as you move.

1. Foundation: Activate and draw muscles from whatever body part is meeting the floor up toward the pelvis. Choices could include, depending on the pose:

Always bend limbs first, to deactivate the outer body more, then:

To establish your hands as a foundation:

- ⁕ root fingertips

- ⁕ press into ring of outer palm of both hands

- ⁕ activate arches of the hand: *hasta bandha*, center of the palm, or "hand support")

- ⁕ lift through inner forearms

- ⁕ Draw inner biceps up toward armpits and then out the back of each shoulder, widening them to the sides in a Y shape.

- ⁕ position the shoulder blades on the back as if standing naturally

- ⁕ soften chest and lower ribs slightly in and up, so they're not jutting out

To establish your feet as a foundation:

- ⁕ ground balls of the feet and heels

- ⁕ lift toes once in a while

- ⁕ activate arches of the feet: *pada bandha,* or "foot support"

- ⁕ lift through the inner shins

- ⁕ firm and draw inner thighs up toward inner groins and then out to widen each sitting bone like a Y-shape.

To establish your pelvis as a foundation:

- ⁕ root sitting bones down firmly.

- ⁕ lengthen pubic bone and tailbone evenly toward the mat

- ⁕ Ground seat and legs into floor if applicable.

2. Core: The central part of your Core Strength Muscle Meridian; made up of the pelvis, sacrum, and lumbar spine.

- Engage and lift the pelvic floor (bathroom muscles) higher, inside the pelvis (pelvic diaphragm) on exhales.

- Release and lower the same areas on inhales.

- Draw front of low-back spine inward and upward. This activates the psoas (pronounced so-as), the dual muscles that run from the upper inner thighs, up the front crests of pelvis, and along the sides of the lumbar spine.

- Draw sacrum and back of the lumbar spine in and up. This activates the quadratus lumborum muscles that run from the rear crest of the pelvis to the sides of lumbar spine and bottom of the back ribs.

3. Expression: The part of the pose that is lifted into length and lightness by the upward-moving work of the Foundation and Core.

- Wave length through the top of the pelvis and lumbar spine to the crown of the head.

- Breathing diaphragm frees for deep breath.

- Tongue activates through Lion's Pose at times.

- Arms lighten and unfurl upward, bending elbows first to root shoulders naturally back.

- Or, if in a Handstand, for example, legs may be the last, highest, lightest point of the pose.

During this program, you'll do a few things differently from the way the majority of yoga is taught.

- **Back off to go deeper:** soften, bend, and begin each pose in a nonlinear way first, instead of rushing toward the full pose.

- **Build every pose from the ground up:** move from Foundation to Core to Expression, always in that order.

- **Move from inner to outer:** activate your Core Strength Muscle Meridian first, instead of overacting from the outer body.

✦ **Go whole:** use your body in a holistic way, not in tension-building parts and pieces.

Don't worry about remembering all of this. Just follow my instructions, and you'll be doing all of this, every time. Use the instructions properly and you'll stimulate your central nervous system in a way that helps you digest, detox, balance, and calm yourself more optimally. Isn't that what we're here for?

You'll get it as you practice, and if needed, I've got everything in video form for you on www.21DayYogaBody.com. So let's move on to the mat!

How to Structure Your Daily Yoga Practice

Do your yoga in this order each day

Use your Belly Bonfire Breath the whole time until you rest at the end.

Start with the Core Warm-Up and Core Sun Salutations.

Do the Daily Core Sequence for that day.

End with the Core Cooldown.

Following are your Everyday Yoga Body Sequences—which are the consistent bookend sequences to your daily practice.

BELLY BONFIRE BREATH

The core of any successful yoga practice is your breath. In fact, integrating breath, intention, and movement is the hallmark of what makes it yoga at all and not, say, Jazzercise.

This breath, like the Wave you'll learn next, is to be done in every available pose, until you're in your final resting posture. Always begin your practice by connecting to your breathing, then add your daily yoga movement to this central focus. I want you to spark a more powerful inner heat as you learn my Belly Bonfire Breath technique. The breath activates all three of your innermost spinal muscular diaphragms—the vocal, breathing, and pelvic diaphragms—and supports the way you're naturally built to breathe. Yogis call these *bandhas* (bun-d'has), which translates to "support" or "lift." We'll use your bandhas in a healing, empowering conversation that will light up the dark inner body—bring new circulation, lymph, and nerve flow there—to help you to detox and optimize cardio, digestion, and reproductive health, too.

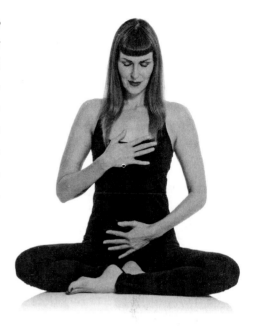

How-To You can learn the breath sitting up in an Easy Seat (see pages 33–34) or on your back in any resting position.

We'll start with a little Ujjayi (oo-*jaii*) Breathing. To do this, you'll need to create resistance at the back of the throat. To find this action at your vocal diaphragm and create the ocean sound that is often used in yoga, do the following:

- ☼ Open your mouth and pretend you're fogging up a window as you sigh out through the mouth.

- ☼ Keep the throat action as you breathe in.

- ☼ Close your lips around the sound, and do this same breath in and out through your nose.

- ☼ If you sound like Darth Vader, that's good. If you sound like you're snoring—that's overkill. Make it audible but smooth.

- ☼ Now turbo-boost it: Close your eyes, and imagine a golden flame sitting in the center and base of your pelvis. GPS it: two inches behind the navel, two inches down.

On Your Inhales

- ☼ Your spine gently lifts deep inside your body, like seaweed rising from the ocean floor.

The Belly Bonfire Breath also tones the pelvic floor diaphragm, which can prevent loss of bladder control and uterine prolapse—and BONUS: it also strengthens orgasms. You're welcome.

- Let the flame warm and widen your pelvis as you relax the muscles of your low belly, pelvic diaphragm, and pelvic floor muscles. Allow your belly to expand down and out like filling up a water balloon—keep your low ribs unmoving and relax the abs instead.

- Imagine torching all that old stuff down there in your "basement" that's holding you back!

- Your inhales are a wave of space from the top of the chest downward to the belly, then pelvis.

On Your Exhales

- Contract the "bathroom" muscles at your pelvic floor, the diamond-shaped area between the sitting bones, pubic bone, and tailbone, and also the higher ones, the ring of muscles inside your pelvic bones.

- Hug them all around that flame, and lift it up behind your navel.

- Your exhales are a wave of inner and outer activation and lift from pelvis to abs to ribs, as if squeezing a tube of toothpaste from the bottom up.

- Think of lifting old tension, stories, and toxins into the fire and burning them away.

Note: If this is a new practice for you, or you've had children, the pelvic diaphragm muscles might be elusive at first. Don't worry—they will build in time, and you will begin to feel them, first subtly and then more clearly.

At first, you might try squeezing the muscles of the more superficial pelvic floor only, like you're trying not to go to the bathroom, but eventually you want to lift the muscular action higher than that. It's like pulling from the diamond of the pelvic floor upward in a pyramid shape into your center pelvis.

The Wave

Core Strength Vinyasa Yoga is, ultimately, a transitional style. Although many styles get you into a pose first and then work alignment, actually, 90 percent of alignment is built before you get into a pose, not after.

As you come into any pose in your practice, don't come up with an overarched back or rigid as a board. Instead, do the Wave up. It's a liquid movement that recruits your Core Strength Muscles, sparing overused outer-body muscles and protecting your spine and joints.

Do the Wave

The Wave travels like this, in this order, every time: Foundation, Core, Expression. Here's how we roll: you'll relax your body toward the floor, then root down, round your back a little, and roll your spine up into every pose.

- Bend and then press your foundation (hands, feet, seat—whatever's on the ground) down firmly to activate the core body.

- Pull your front hips and spine in and upward to support the natural low-back curve.

- Begin to roll up, relaxing the upper body. Add the natural low-back curve.

- Wave your spine long from the centered pelvis out through your head.

- Let your arms—or whatever's lifting—bend and unroll up into your Expression.

In time, when you learn to do the Wave more smoothly, it will become second nature in all your poses—or better, first nature.

CORE WARM-UP

Do Flow 1 at least 3 times through. Do Flow 2 at least 3 to 5 times through as fast or slow as you wish. Include a Vinyasa (see pages 41-43) after any Down Dog or where it feels appropriate, or skip it and just rest in a Dog pose or Child's Pose for 5 breaths.

FLOW 1: FIRE UP THE CORE

Easy Seat Rollup

- ❋ Sit on a yoga block at the front of your mat with one foot placed in front of the other—no crossed ankles.

- ❋ From this seat, reach your arms forward to the floor, and take 5 breaths here.

- ❋ Roll back up to sit, feeling your sitting bones press (Foundation), your front pelvis and low back drawing in and up evenly (Core), and your spine, chest, arms, and head lightening and lengthening upward (Expression).

 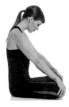 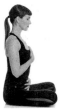

Repeat these rollups 5 times.

Core Dedication

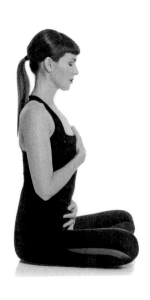

- ❋ In your Easy Seat, rest one palm on your heart center, not your actual heart! The yogi "heart" of good lovin' energy is inside the middle of your chest.

- ❋ Place the other palm on your lower belly.

Do your Belly Bonfire Breath for at least 1 minute:

- ❋ Inhales relax your belly and pelvis.

- ❋ Exhales hug and lift from pelvis to belly to ribs.

- ❋ As you breathe, remember your Core Inspiration today. Keep it in mind as you move through each pose. Slowly open your eyes, and move on to the Seated Spinal Arch/Curl.

Seated Spinal Arch/Curl

- Place your hands on your knees.

- Inhale deeply through your nose, lean forward, and then arch your chest upward.

- Exhale, round your back. Keep your low back long here. Stretch the back of your chest upward to release upper-back tension.

Repeat Seated Spinal Arch/Curls 5 to 10 times.

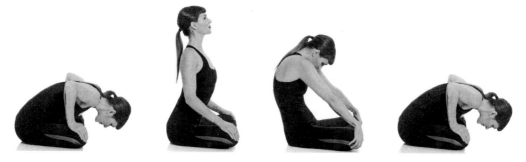

Fists of Fire Crossed-Ankle Boat Pose

- Next, inhale in Easy Seat, reach your arms overhead. Rock back onto your sitting bones, sit up tall, and lift your knees toward your chest, shins and feet parallel to the floor. Bring fists into your hips.

- Rock forward into Easy Seat, arms up.

- Exhale, rock back into Crossed-Ankle Boat with Fists of Fire.

Repeat Fists of Fire Crossed-Ankle Boat Pose 5 times.

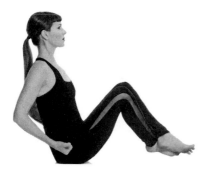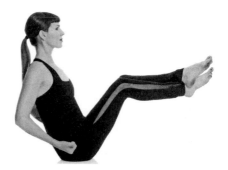

Scissor Kick

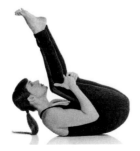

- ⁖ Place forearms down on the floor behind you.

- ⁖ Bend your knees, and lift them up over your hip joints.

  - ⁖ Inhale.

  - ⁖ Exhale, kick your left leg out long through the heel as you draw your right knee closer to the chest. Yell "Ha!" to detox stress and energize the solar plexus.

  - ⁖ Maintain the lift through your low back so that you're not collapsing.

  - ⁖ Inhale, and return both knees over hips.

  - ⁖ Exhale, and kick out through the right heel.

Repeat Scissor Kicks 10 to 20 times on each side.

Rock 'n' Roll Pose

- ⁖ Hug your knees to your chest. Hang on behind your knees.

- ⁖ Roll down onto your back, massaging each vertebra as you go.

- ⁖ Exhale, and roll up into Boat Pose: knees bent and feet lifted off the floor.

- ⁖ Sitting bones root down strongly to wave the spine higher and lift the chest.

Repeat Rock 'n' Roll Pose into Boat Pose 3 to 5 times. Then hold Boat Pose for 3 breaths.

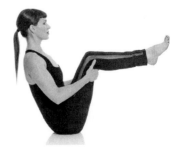

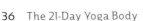

Goddess Boat Pose

⁖ Bring your hands together in Charlie's Angels Mudra (a fun yet intentional hand position, otherwise known as the Venus Mudra for empowerment): all fingers interlace except your pointed index fingers, which join together.

⁖ Stretch your arms out long in front of you.

⁖ Place your feet together on the floor.

⁖ Inhale, widen your knees, and open the soles of the feet like a book as you lean forward and reach your arms farther out. Stretch the inner thigh meridian.

⁖ Exhale, keep your arms pointing forward and plank your long torso back; lean back as if in a Boat Pose but with your knees widened and lifted closer to your chest.

Repeat Goddess Boat Pose 3 to 5 times.

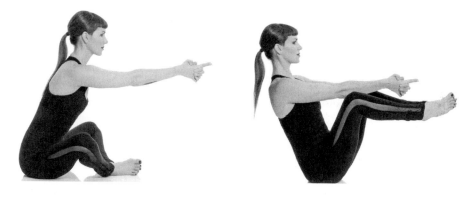

After your last Goddess Boat Pose, cross your ankles and either step or press hands down, lift your belly, and hop back into Downward-Facing Dog.

Downward-Facing Dog

Before you step back and put pressure on the wrists, align your hands now to protect the wrists in a more open state.

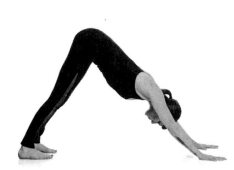

- ❖ Put your knees down for a moment.

  - ❖ Plant your hands shoulder-distance apart at the front of your mat. Do a shoulder-to-wrist check, and make sure you're not placing the hands too close or too wide.

  - ❖ Turn your middle fingers to face forward out of a wrist crease that's parallel to the front of your mat, not twisted in or out.

  - ❖ Lift one, then the other hand onto Spidey fingertips only. Slide and press down from fingertips to palm again until hands are flat but superhero—grounding!

- ❖ Press the fingertips and ring of your palm down strongly. You want to feel the inner palm lift upward. This is your core strength waking up.

- ❖ Tuck your toes under, and lift your knees and hips into the pose.

DOWN DOG WAVE

Often students have too much back arch, dropped shoulders, and compressed joints in this pose. Let's give our Dog a treat with a luscious Wave to decompress and realign the spine:

- ❖ Lift your heels upward to activate and integrate the legs.

- ❖ Pull in your belly and ribs to round your back and shoulders upward. Make sure you have armpits, the sign of healthy shoulder joints!

- ❖ Wave length through your spine from up here so that it moves longer through the crown.

- ❖ Slide your shoulder blades down the back naturally.

- ❖ Press equally back down through your heels, even as you try to lift them up. Sounds like I hopped on the Crazy Train just then, but this way, you will actually get a nice activated lengthening instead of a passive overstretch.

Hold your new, decompressed Down Dog for 3 to 5 breaths.

Diabloasana

- ✢ From Down Dog, come down onto your hands and knees.

- ✢ Place your forearms onto the mat with your shoulders stacked above your elbows.

- ✢ Interlace your fingers.

- ✢ Press through the arms, lift your top front pelvis and front low-back spine firmly away from the mat. Your tailbone will lengthen and your belly will tone.

- ✢ Walk your feet back until legs are straight, knees are off the floor.

- ✢ Press back through your heels strongly to firm the legs.

- ✢ You're now in a Plank-like pose with forearms down.

- ✢ Place your knees down if your belly and hips are sagging, but keep lifting up the deep psoas-activated core.

- ✢ Exhale, and spin both heels to the left. This will twist your legs to the right.

- ✢ Keep your chest and arms centered as you tone your side body and core.

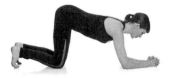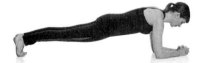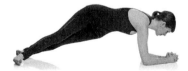

- ✢ Inhale back to center.

- ✢ Exhale; heels drop to the right, legs spin to the left.

- Inhale, center.
- If your knees need to come down, just tilt the hips over to one side and then the other.

Repeat Diabloasana 3 to 5 times.

Child's Pose

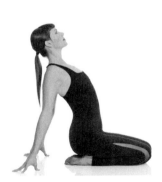

- Put the knees down.
- Press your hips back to your heels and fold forward, forehead on the floor or a block.
- Knees come together if you want more of a low-back and sacrum stretch, or widen them with big toes touching for a belly release, groin, and inner-thigh opening.
- Relax your arms forward or back, or give a detoxing massage with fists into your low belly.

Breathe in Child's Pose for 5 to 10 breaths.

Vargasasana

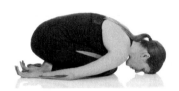

- Begin to roll up to sit.
- Walk your fingertips behind you, facing forward.
- Draw your front spine in and up as you arch your chest upward to stretch the shoulders, chest, and belly.
- Keep your neck curve long and natural; just look slightly up. Imagine an orange behind your neck; in yoga poses, you never want to drop the skull back and make orange juice.
- Draw your shoulders back more, and press firmly down into the hands.

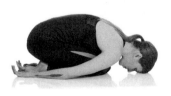

Take 3 to 5 breaths here. Return to Child's Pose for 1 to 3 breaths to counterpose. Repeat Flow 1 1 to 3 times, then continue to Flow 2: Core Sun Salutations.

FLOW 2: CORE SUN SALUTATIONS

First: Learn the Core Vinyasa Sequence

Why: The Core Vinyasa, or centered flow, is my anatomical redesign of a traditional in-between sequence that you can insert after any Down Dog or between standing pose sequences to amp up the intensity of your practice. You can do it a lot or skip it whenever you want. Take one breath or more in each pose, but try to transition to the next pose on an exhale first as you begin moving, then an inhale to fill the pose once you arrive. This will ensure more support for your low back as you move.

My updated version will get and keep you optimally safe and strong as you move from pose to pose.

Dog to Core Plank Wave

- ❖ Come into Down Dog. This is different from the Dog Wave: now we're going to flow into a stronger pose.

- ❖ Bend your knees and lift the heels.

- ❖ Exhale; lift your belly and roll forward into the top of a push-up: your front, top hip crests pull inward, the front lumbar spine and ribs lift as you round the back forward until shoulders stack straight over the hands.

- ❖ Think of leading with the back of your chest as you pull forward.

- ❖ Inhale and add the sacrum and low back curving in and up to lengthen through the front chest and crown of the head.

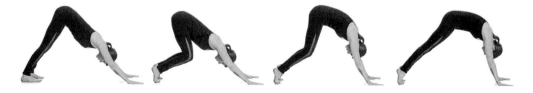

- Don't lose the strong tone of the front pelvic crests and front spine or you'll hang out in the low back too much here.

- Beginners: put your knees down in this pose whenever needed.

Half or Full Chaturanga (chaht-oor-ahn-gah)

- Place your knees down in Plank Pose if needed.

- Inhale, and shift your heels and chest forward as you bend your elbows over wrists.

- Lift your front spine into your body.

- Lower 1 inch or more, moving toward a low, floating push-up.

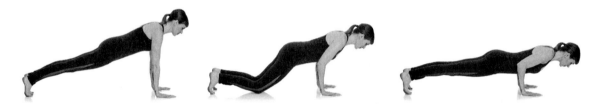

It's best not to aim for a perfect "halfway down" position in this pose. Anytime your shoulders dip lower than your elbow joints, it causes massive strain. Instead, as I'm doing here, hover higher than your elbows and you'll build muscle, not pressure.

To check your alignment, put a yoga block halfway up your mat and rest your hips on it as you lower to Chaturanga.

Cobra or Upward-Facing Dog

- Lower your hips to the mat. Keep your shoulders up on the back.

- Point your toes and press your feet into the floor.

- Exhale, push your hands down strongly, and use the momentum to round your back first. This counteracts an overarching low back.

- Unroll the chest open, leading with the back of your chest and back skull, moving back and up—not jutting out your chest.

- You can remain in Baby Cobra (with ribs still on the mat) or, if it feels good, lift the torso up a little higher, just your hips and legs remaining on the floor, for Teenage Cobra.

- Inhale here to fill the chest and belly.

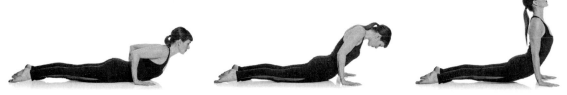

If you can go higher, move into Upward-Facing Dog instead of Cobra.

- Come into a higher arch as you straighten your arms more.

- Your collarbones are parallel to the ground and your front thighs lightly brush the floor.

- Slide your head back and up without lifting your chin much—remember: no orange juice.

- Inhale in your full Expression.

Transition from Cobra to Up Dog

To get back to Dog with no lower-back strain, you have two options:

KNEE-DOWN PLANK

- Exhale, press knees down into the mat,

- The hands ground down as your front pelvis (psoas) pulls you upward and back into Down Dog pose.

- Step your feet over from pointed to balls of the feet as you move into the pose.

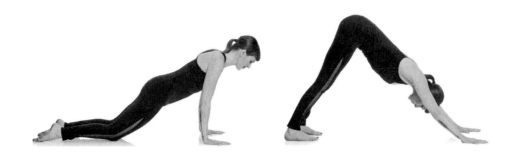

Work toward this stronger variation to totally tone the deeper core muscles:

POINTED PLANK

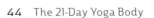

⁘ From your Cobra or Up Dog, keep your toes pointed.

⁘ Exhale, press hands into the floor strongly as your legs, front hips, and spine all lift up in one line so that you're in a Plank on the tops of your pointed feet.

⁘ Continue sending hips up and back, as one foot and then the other steps over into Down Dog.

Hold Down Dog for 3 to 5 breaths here.

Down Dog to Lunge

⁘ In Downward-Facing Dog, keep your hips square.

⁘ Inhale, and lift the right leg up.

⁘ Flex through your heel, and keep the leg strong.

⁘ Draw lightly up the front of the body to resist arching your back or dropping out through the shoulders.

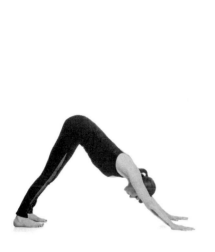
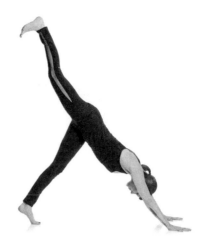

Move into Core Plank

This pose teaches you to use physics power to gain core power and lightness. So you really need to bend your arms!

∗• Begin to bend both elbows straight back and hug them in to line up the forearms as if you're about to take your parallel forearms to the floor. Wrist creases should now be centered forward.

∗• Bend your standing leg, too.

∗• As you exhale, simultaneously
  • Press your arms and standing leg straight.
  • Use the momentum rising up from the earth to round your back high and sweep your right knee into your chest.
  • Move shoulders forward over wrists.
  • Inhale back to Dog Splits.

Repeat this move 1 to 3 times, and then on your last exhale:

∗• From the high hips and chest, lightly step the right foot to the right thumb, not between the hands. This places the foot in line with your hip joint.

∗• You're now in a Low Lunge pose.

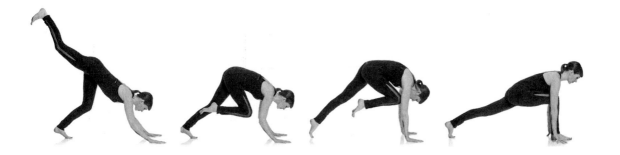

Come into Fists of Fire Lunge

꘠ Exhale, root your feet strongly, and lift your front pelvis away from the front thigh.

꘠ Keep your arms completely relaxed and hanging down.

꘠ Begin to roll up over your legs, drawing front pelvis in and up.

꘠ Then draw in your sacrum and low-back curve.

꘠ As the momentum hits your chest, bend elbows up and unfurl your arms to the sky. This lessens the load on the upper back and shoulder muscles, which can build tension, not strength.

꘠ Reach up for a breath or two here in High Lunge.

Come into Fists of Fire High Lunge

꘠ Inhale in High Lunge.

꘠ Exhale, bend your back knee, and sweep both hands into fists down beside your hips.

꘠ Take this opportunity to re-center your pelvis and lower belly in and up.

꘠ Inhale, and reach arms up again.

Repeat Fists of Fire High Lunge 3 to 5 times.

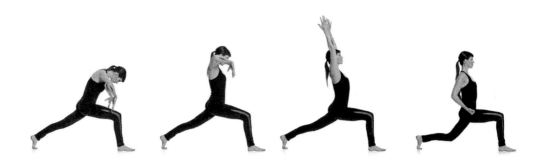

Move into Fierce Lion Lunge

From your last fists-into-hips position

- Inhale, and lean your torso more forward over your front leg.

- Reach arms long by your ears.

- Exhale, sweep fists into Fists of Fire position, and then keep going, as you open your fingers behind you and think of "letting go" of what no longer serves your core strength.

- As you do this, stick your tongue out, and roar like a lion! Haaaa! That's superfierce.

Repeat Fierce Lion Lunge 3 to 5 times or until you laugh.

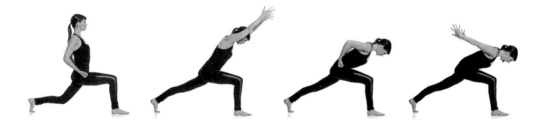

On an exhale, return your hands to the mat, and step back into Downward-Facing Dog.

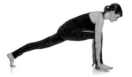 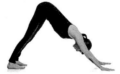

Shakti Kicks (optional)

⁖ From your last Dog pose, walk both feet together. Press the big toe mounds into the mat and keep your feet magnetized like this for the whole pose.

⁖ Inhale, lift your heels, and bend both knees.

⁖ Bend your elbows straight back, too, as if in Core Plank preparation.

⁖ Exhale, and simultaneously press your hands down, arms straightening.

⁖ Use that momentum, plus a firm Belly Bonfire exhale/pelvic lift, to raise the pelvis higher as you jump, and try to kick your own sitting bones with both your heels.

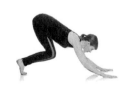 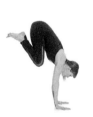 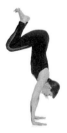

⁖ Land back in the first position with bent knees. Then inhale, prepare.

⁖ Exhale, kick again!

Try 3 to 5 Shakti Kicks, and then on your last exhale:

❖ Pretend to jump over something lying right in the middle of your mat to get your pelvis and feet lifting higher as you hop your feet between your hands.

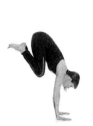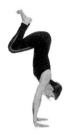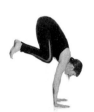

If you can't hop all the way forward in one hop, then hop-walk or walk up; but as you can, chip away at this move by hopping, even one inch forward—you'll get stronger and more courageous every time.

Spinal Wave to Forward Fold

❖ On a few breaths or, ultimately, on a single inhale, wave your spine forward—but from your Foundation first:

- Press your feet down and lift your toes to activate the Deep Core Line arches.
- Keep your knees a little bent.
- Pull your lower belly upward and your front low-back spine away from the thighs. This is almost a rounding of your back that helps you access your psoas and support the low-back spine, which many people overarch here.
- Wave your spine and the crown of your head long from the pelvis.

❖ Exhale, fold over your still-charged legs for Forward Fold. Don't jam your legs straight. Instead, play your edge, and invite your body to open slowly over the course of your entire practice.

Try it again:

❖ Inhale, and lift your low belly up and over your legs.

❖ Exhale, and cascade your spine and head even farther down.

Breathe in your Forward Fold for 1 to 5 breaths.

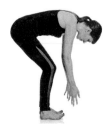 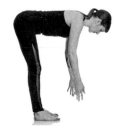 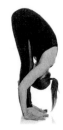

Roll into Mountain Pose

- Inhale, bend your knees, and prepare.

- Exhale; hug and lift your Golden Flame pelvic muscles as you begin to press your feet down and roll up to stand. This protects your lumbar spine as you come up, and you won't get as dizzy.

- Once the pelvis is stacked over legs, inhale; as you continue up, arms unroll to the sky from the lifting spine.

- Exhale, and bring palms together at the chest.

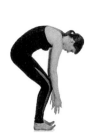 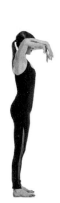 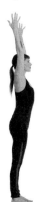 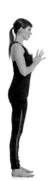

Flow Back into Downward-Facing Dog

- Bend your knees a little in Mountain Pose.

- Exhale, press feet down, and ripple a wave upward through your legs, pelvis, spine, and arms.

- Inhale, reach arms to the sky.

- Exhale, bend your knees, and fold into Forward Fold.

- Straighten the legs to your healthy edge here.

- Inhale, and take a Spinal Wave into a long back. Look forward!

- Exhale, plant your hands, and step back into Downward-Facing Dog pose.

    Take a Vinyasa, Fists of Fire, and Fierce Lion Lunge on your other side. Repeat your Core Sun Salutation 3 to 5 times through on each side. Rest in Child's Pose whenever needed.

DAILY CORE COOLDOWN SEQUENCE

I crafted this specific ending flow for you to do directly after you finish your creative sequence every day to ensure that you gain the most benefits from all your efforts on the mat. You will stretch and detox your whole body plus release excess tension from the Core Strength Muscle Meridian. Stretching makes your muscles leaner and keeps them from limiting your range of motion. So don't skip it to go check your e-mail. Your Yoga Body will thank you!

FLOW 1: STARGAZER FLOW

Pigeon Pose

- Come into Downward-Facing Dog. Lift your right leg.

- Exhale through Core Plank, and place your right knee behind the right wrist.

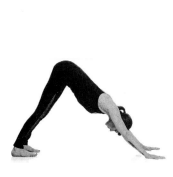
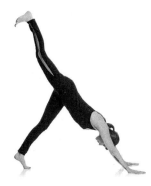
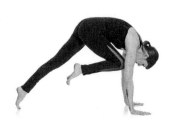

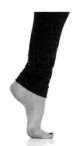

:• Lengthen your back leg straight out behind you, foot pointed on the floor.

:• Center your hips forward.

:• Your front foot is in Stilettoasana (pointed through the ball of the foot, with the toes pulled back as if you were wearing high heels). This will help the foot and shin roll open more easily and protect the knee from torque as you fold.

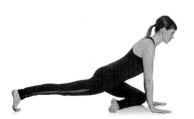
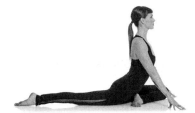

:• Widen the front knee to point straight out of or, if comfortable, wider than the front hip joint.

Do not grab your foot or flex the foot here to avoid twisting your knee as you come back to center. To deepen the stretch, keep your pelvis evenly forward, slide your front knee open more, and creep your back leg back.

:• Begin to walk your hands back as you roll up from the floor: pull the lower belly in and up, and contain the lower ribs.

:• Breathe here. Keep hips centering.

- Exhale, and fold forward, forearms on a block or the floor.

- Rest your head on your hands or a block for calming.

Take 5 to 10 or more slow, gentle breaths here.

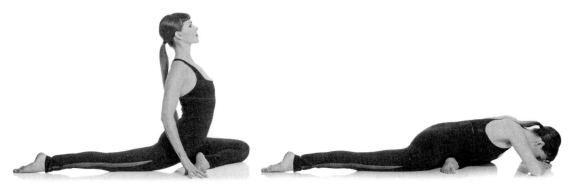

PIGEON POSE TO JANU SIRSASANA
(JAHN-OO SEER-SHAH-SUH-NUH)

- Swing your back leg around until it faces straight forward and you're sitting fully on your sitting bones.

- Bend your left foot into the right inner thigh. Foot is still in Stilet-toasana.

- Flex your other foot through the heel; firm the leg into the mat.

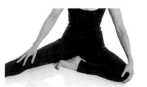

- Plant your fingertips on the floor behind you as you inhale and wave the spine long.

- Exhale, and begin to lean your torso and head forward in one long line. Press your fingertips back to help you fold.

Avoid the tendency to round your back and lead with your face. Sit up tall, and you'll get a more holistic back-body stretch even if you don't go as far down.

- Feel free to walk your hands forward to frame your leg or shin, and eventually, you might even take hold of the right foot.

- Ground both sitting bones evenly.

- Inhale, and lift your belly up and over the leg.

- Exhale, and fold deeper.

Take 5 to 10 breaths here.

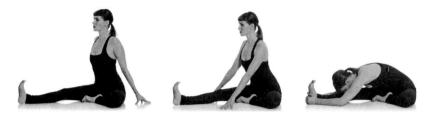

SIDE JANU SIRSASANA

- Stay low in your fold, but do the following:

- Place your right elbow inside your right knee. Bend the leg if needed.

- Inhale, and lengthen your spine.

- Exhale, and twist the chest and shoulders open to the left, in a side-bend position, opening your left hip and knee farther back if you want.

- Side bend over your right leg.

- You might place your bottom forearm on the floor, walk the hand farther forward, or even hook the elbow inside the knee and grab your foot.

- Rest your head in the bottom hand's fingertips so that you can relax the neck muscles but keep opening your chest to the left.

- Unroll your top arm with a bent elbow; then reach the arm over the top ear.

- To get a delicious stretch in your QL (quadratus lumborum, a deep lumbar muscle running from back hips to back low ribs), root your left hip down more, and stretch away from it with the left, top hand.

- Soften your outer side waist muscles, and let the stretch move deeper toward the spine.

Take 5 to 10 breaths in Side Janu Sirsasana.

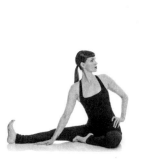
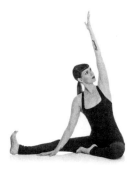
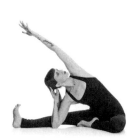

Stargazer

- ❖ Exhale, come up to sit, chest still facing open to the left.

- ❖ Place your left hand behind your left hip, flat palm, middle finger facing the back of your mat.

- ❖ Press into your hand, and roll onto the front of your left shin as you lift your hips off the mat.

- ❖ Draw the lower belly in and up to lengthen the tailbone, and sweep your right arm over your ear, or place the hand behind your head for support.

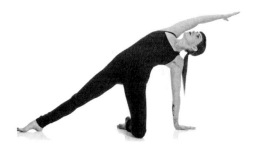

- ❖ Press your long neck and skull back to reveal this juicy, heart-opening pose.

  Be here for 1 to 5 breaths.

  Return to Downward-Facing Dog. Repeat Flow 1 on your other side.

FLOW 2: SPINAL STRETCH AND DETOX

Seated Forward Fold

- ❖ Sit up evenly on your sitting bones.

- ❖ Stretch both legs out in front of you, feet flexed back.

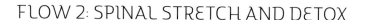

- Plant your fingertips behind you, and engage your legs into the floor.

- Inhale, and wave the spine long from sitting bones to crown.

- Exhale, hinge at your hip creases, and fold—don't round—forward. Continue to sweep your low-back curve in and up.

- Back your head off in line with your spine, and let the chest lead the way.

- Inhale, and scoop your lower belly up and over your pelvis more.

- Exhale and fold.

Remain in Seated Forward Fold for 5 to 10 breaths.

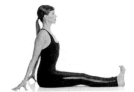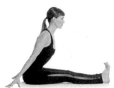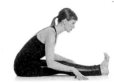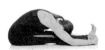

When you're finished, come back to sit. Bend your knees. Reach your arms forward for balance, and roll slowly onto your back.

Bridge Pose Preparation and Bridge Pose

- Bend your knees, feet on the mat.

- Walk your feet back until they plant under the knees, just in front of the sitting bones.

- Arms press into the mat beside hips, palms down.

- Inhale, prepare.

- Exhale, and lift your hips up as if you have a supportive hand under your sacrum—no crunching the lower back.

- Draw your front lumbar spine in to counterbalance the curve.

- At first, leave your arms as they are to breathe into the back of your chest and lungs.

- Then roll your shoulders underneath you more, and interlace your fingers or clasp palms. Breathe into your front and upper chest here.

- Avoid pushing your collarbones away from your ears too much.

- Lift your chin, and slide the back of your head toward your body so that your neck curve stays natural. You should be able to slide a hand underneath your neck and not flatten it into the floor.

Breathe in Bridge Pose for 5 to 10 breaths.

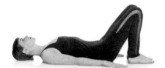 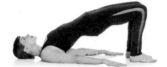 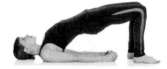

Full Wheel

This is an optional, more advanced backbend. Try it, but be mindful.

- Bend your elbows, and place your hands next to your ears with fingers pointing back toward your shoulders.

- Aim to gently hug elbows in toward hand width, like Chaturanga alignment. Root your shoulder blades onto the back and firmly down, to avoid disengaging your arm strength.

- Inhale, prepare.

- Exhale, firm your Golden Flame pelvic muscles to anchor the sacrum, and draw down into your front lumbar spine as you press hands and feet to come up into the backbend.

- In the pose, lift your heels up for more freedom in your lower back.

- Lift your pubic bone upward, but activate a Deep Core Line wave that draws your top, front pelvic crests, front lumbar, lower ribs, and skull toward the back body more; then lengthen the whole spine through the crown. This should free your lower back from compression and make this a backbend, not a forward jut.

Breathe here for 3 to 5 breaths; then bend your elbows, tuck your chin to come slowly down onto your shoulder blades, and roll your hips back onto the mat.

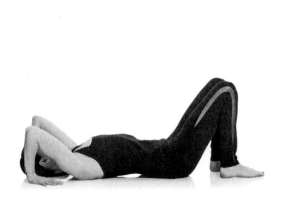
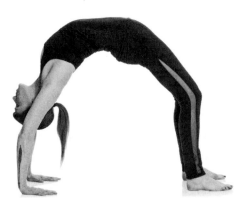

Move into Sacral Reset Pose

- Grab your yoga block.

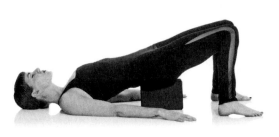

- Lift your hips, and place the block the long way, so it sets right into the sacrum at the center of your back pelvis, not your lower back.

- Scoot your head and shoulders a few inches away from the block so that you get more spinal traction in your lower back curve here and your sacrum resets deeper into the pelvis.

Then take one, or more, of the following three variations:

SACRUM STRETCH

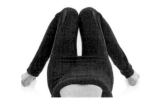

> ∴ Walk your feet as wide as your mat, and let your knees relax in toward each other. They don't have to touch. This move will open tight muscles around the sacrum.

> ∴ Reach your arms overhead on the floor if you like.

PSOAS RELEASE

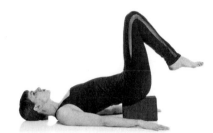

> ∴ Walk your feet together, and lift your bent knees into the air to hover right over your hips.

> ∴ Totally relax your legs and feet here.

SUPPORTED SHOULDER STAND

A classical shoulder stand runs the risk of compressing and flattening the neck spine. Instead, try this variation that gives you the same full-body detoxing inversion benefits without the possible negative side effects.

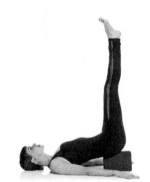

> ∴ From your Psoas Release position, straighten your legs into the air over your hips and block. Turn the block the wider way if you need more balance support.

> **Breathe in your variation(s) for 1 to 5 minutes.**

When done, lower the feet back into Bridge prep, lift hips, remove the block, and roll slowly down to the mat. Enjoy your new, spacious sacrum and low back. Move on to Flow 3.

FLOW 3: LEG RESET TO FINAL REST

Scissor Stretch

> ∴ Hug your right knee into your chest. The left leg can stay bent or lengthen onto the mat.

> ∴ Interlace the fingers of both hands behind the center of your right thigh.

- Straighten your leg up to a 90-degree angle.

- Press your hands and thigh together, and activate up through the heel as you deepen your groins toward the floor.

Take 5 breaths here.

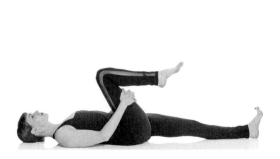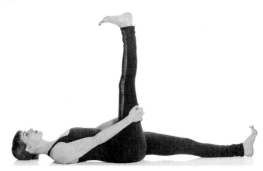

IT Stretch

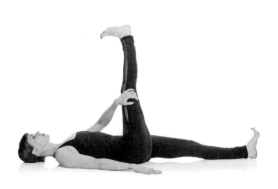

- Switch your left hand to the outside of the right thigh; place your right hand on the floor or hook the right thumb into your right hip crease and press the thigh away from your pelvis to traction the joint and spine.

- Begin to angle your lifted leg 15 degrees or so over to the left. Keep your right hip down to get the best stretch along the outer side (IT band) of your right leg.

Take 5 breaths here.

Half Happy Baby Pose

- Bend the right knee and hang on to your right shin, inner knee, or ball of the foot. Keep your pelvis flat on the floor.

- Option: straighten the leg open to the side for Half Reclining Fan Pose (a great inner-thigh stretch).

Take 5 to 10 breaths.

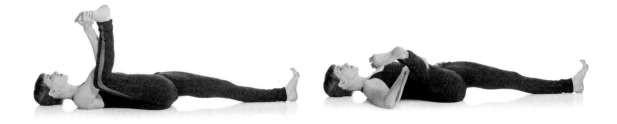

Eagle Twist

- Widen the arms into a T on the mat.

- Cross your bent left knee over your right knee.

- If you can, wrap the left shin, and maybe the foot, around the right leg.

- Scoot just your hips (not the shoulders) over to the left side of your mat.

- Drop your knees gently to the right.

- Let your head roll to the left.

- No need to yank your legs here—the lower back is not supposed to twist deeply. Just relax and breathe.

Be in Eagle Twist for 5 breaths. Repeat the sequence from Scissor Stretch on the other leg, then continue to Full Happy Baby Pose.

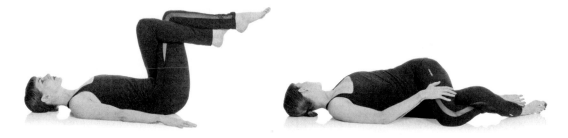

Full Happy Baby Pose

❧ Come onto your back.

❧ Bend both knees. Hold on to both shins or outer feet.

❧ Keep your pelvis flat—your hips should not roll up off the floor.

❧ Rock from side to side and/or lengthen both legs out into Full Reclining Fan Pose and stretch those inner thighs.

Take 5 to 10 breaths here.

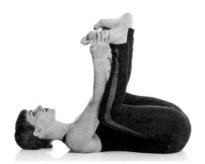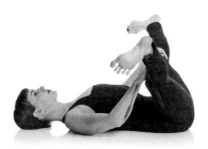

Reclining Goddess

❧ Lower your legs to the floor. Bring the balls of your feet together, and open your knees to the side for Reclining Goddess.

❧ If your knees are way off the floor or you feel a strain in your groins here, place a block or pillow under each outer knee.

❧ Rest one palm on your heart, one on your lower belly.

Breathe very slowly and gently for 1 to 5 minutes here, and as you do:

❧ Inhale to create more space in the chest, belly, and pelvis. Make space for your inner energy to expand more fully into your skin.

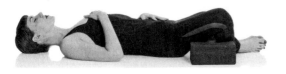

❧ Exhale, let go, and allow gravity to cleanse away the breath and wash away any old, limiting beliefs or actions that no longer serve your greatness.

Spinal Traction Pose

- Keep the knees bent, and place your feet back down into a Bridge Pose Preparation.

- With legs still bent, place your palms onto your upper thighs right before they meet the hip creases. The closer you are to the root of your legs, the better this will feel.

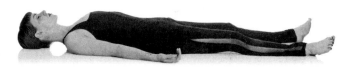

- Press your thighs away gently but firmly with your hands, and relax your legs, hips, and lower back.

- This should bring a feeling of stretch and space into your pelvis and lumbar spine.

  Take 3 to 5 breaths here.

Final Resting Pose—Savasana
(shuh-vah-sah-nah)

- Stretch your legs out, and come to rest on your back completely.

- Slide your shoulder blades naturally down your back, and tuck your tailbone lightly underneath you.

- Stretch your arms and legs away from the torso more, and scoot your skull away from your shoulders a little.

- Take a big breath into your chest, expand the belly, and fill your whole body with more energy and life.

- Exhale through your mouth, sigh it out, and relax even more deeply into the floor, as if making an impression down into warm sand.

- Release the valve in your throat, and breathe naturally through the nose or mouth. Listen attentively for your inner wisdom and inspiration to speak to you when it's ready, and allow the practice to work its magic on all levels.

You'll hold this pose a bit longer than most, so it can fully cool down your fascia, and reset your body into a new, transformed shape. Lying down in this position creates an awesome alignment of your body—the perfect position to seal yourself into.

Resist the urge to get up—it takes about 3 to 5 minutes to cool the mold. While you're here, watch that you don't begin time traveling with your mind to the anxiety-causing past or future. Turn your curiosity inward, and be right where you are, with high-quality presence.

Contemplate your moment intimately as if it were a sleeping lover's face: What sounds are there? What sensations? Observe them all from your calm center, and float in unhurried awareness for a while. Rest and restore for 3 to 5 minutes here.

Core Sealing Sequence

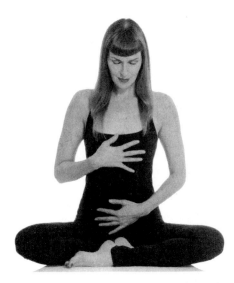

- ✷ After Final Rest, roll to your right side in a fetal position; relax here.

- ✷ Slowly roll yourself up to an Easy Seat, moving through Foundation, Core, and Expression.

- ✷ Place one hand on your belly and the other on your heart center.

- ✷ Take a big inhale, down to the inner flame that lights your own heart from the inside.

- ✷ Exhale, and bow forward, sealing your practice into your deepest center.

Congratulations! You've made it to the mat today—and rocked it. Namaste.

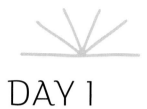

DAY 1

THEME: Find Your Balance

Many people strive for 100 percent vitality, happiness, and peace, removing huge swaths of food from their diet; or aim to cut out every speck of drama from their lives. This can actually cause no end of irritation, dissatisfaction, and all-around frustration. Anyone who has vowed to never eat french fries ever again and then Hungry Hippoed an entire plate of the ones that his or her unsuspecting date ordered knows this to be true.

When you aim for only the good feelings and don't allow any discomfort or imperfection—two places where wisdom, growth, and transformation often happen—the opposite of freedom occurs.

Why has your quest for pie-in-the-sky balance turned you into a control freak? We have confused balance with symmetry, superglued over the heart-wrenching beauty of our grand design with a one-size-fits-all mentality.

In fact, the more I practice yoga and dance with this wild, wacky flow of balance, the more I realize that the idea of some static center—where if we all work hard enough, are popular or lucky enough, we earn our ticket to la-la land for the rest of our days—is a dangerous myth. Seeking happiness over empowerment can diminish both.

And, paradoxically, the more you let go of the strain of seeking unnatural symmetry disguised as balance and allow the dance of center to interweave your life, the better you will physically feel inside and out, the more your mind will relax, and the more success you'll be able to create. Which, of course, brings you closer to that "woo-hoo!" feeling of living life from your core.

This is center: you, a bathing suit, an inner tube, a beer, a perfect summer day, floating down a creek with no paddles and not a care for how long it will take you to arrive.

If, however, you insist on death-gripping onto symmetry, you will become more obsessive, controlling, rigid, and not very fun to be around—for others or for you, who lives here 24-7.

Is your inner space a welcoming world or a world of hurt? How stressful would it be to try to force linear perfection on, say, a passionate tango? The fun of seeking balance is not to aim for a frozen, wax-museum existence. It's to get conscious, every day, find the places where you feel most alive . . . then dance.

So if you really want to find balance, then you have to drop the hard grip on something you've been trying to control and get busy living out loud and access your inner reservoir of core strength and wisdom. And guess what? This is going to look more like eighty-twenty than fifty-fifty or God forbid, 100 percent.

The eighty-twenty rule means that around 80 percent of the time, you are invested in living, loving, eating, moving, thinking, and taking actions that nourish you and bring you more into balance. The remaining 20 percent of the time you might fall off the healthy, empowered, and balance-seeking wagon, and that's just fine.

The first step along any path to reclaiming your whole self is to move from the end of the line back to the middle path. This is truly the road less traveled. Let's explore it together.

YOGA

On and off the mat, often our expression of balance is actually a compressed symmetry. Whenever you come into a pose with straight limbs and an overarched, tight lower back, you've said sayonara to balance, helloooo, symmetry.

Man-made things are the only perfectly symmetrical things. Nature is perfectly balanced.

Have you ever seen a tree that is made of totally straight lines? That would be freakier than the *Blair Witch Project*. A tree is twisty, gnarled, magnificent in its design, as is a river, a sunflower, and, dear reader, you.

Your bones are built in spirals. Your blood and breath moves in spirals. Your whole natural existence is a spiral, circle, and wave. There is no straight line in your whole being. To aim for a strait-laced way of life is to bind yourself into an unnatural shape, and this will strain your mind, heart, and spirit.

You exist in balance, not symmetry. And, baby . . . it's time to get wild.

Today you will begin to solidify your Foundation, the first step toward finding your centermost Core Strength; then you'll wave up from there. As you move through your yoga sequence, apply the eighty-twenty rule to the experience of being on your mat. Strong but expressive should replace linear. Curiosity and sensitivity are more powerful aims than reaching any goal.

As you learn to root down into your bones—which are your foundational points—in a specific way that ignites the soft tissues of *hasta bandha* (arch support of the hands) and *pada bandha* (arch support of the feet), you will begin to activate your Core Strength Muscle Meridian most effectively. From there, build the posture with grace. Let the process of balance unfold.

Begin with 3 to 5 rounds of your Core Warm-Up.

Climb the Mountain

You'll create a wave from the rooting feet rolling upward through the pelvis and lumbar, expressing into a lighter upper body and arms. It's elemental to work your balance from the ground up!

Welcome to your new yoga practice! Remember, I've made you videos of each sequence online at www.21DayYogaBody .com, if you find it easier to follow that way.

- Come to stand at the front of your mat, feet hip-joint-distance apart (this is the width of two fists between the arches of your feet).

- Bend your knees deeply, and slowly roll down until your relaxed hands puddle on the floor.

- Press the balls and heels of both feet downward, and lift your toes to engage the arches.

- Exhale; roll up slowly to stand. You'll get less dizzy and protect your lower back.

- Inhale as you bend your elbows (to release tight shoulders) and unroll your arms effortlessly overhead.

- Exhale, roll down again.

Repeat this Mountain Roll 5 to 10 times.

Open Arms Lunge

This one is named for one of my favorite road trip bands, Journey.

- From Mountain Roll, step your left foot back into a High Lunge; front spine in and up, arms reach up.

- Maintain strong feet as legs and hips square forward.

- Inhale, and lengthen your spine.

- Exhale, spin your chest to the right, and open your arms to the sides.

- Spend a few breaths here, waving the spine long on the inhales, spinning a bit more, and perhaps looking to the right as you exhale. Aim to anchor your legs and pelvis forward, and don't twist into the lower back but only from the chest and higher.

- Then circle: Inhale, sweep your back arm down, forward, and up back into High Lunge. Exhale, open it into Open Arms Lunge again.

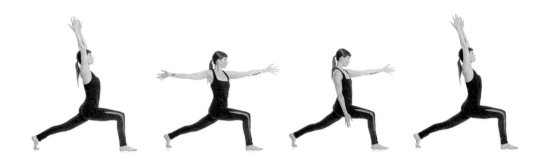

Repeat 3 to 5 times. On your last circle into High Lunge, lean forward, and try to balance on your right foot as you transition into Eagle Pose.

Eagle Pose

- Root the right foot down, and lift the left knee.

- Cross the left knee over the right knee.

- Wrap the foot outside or inside of the right shin.

- Activate your inner thighs into groins and out through the sitting bones, and draw your front lumbar spine in and up to stabilize from overcurving or tipping the pelvis too far forward.

- Lift arms, and place your right elbow onto the inner crease of the left elbow.

- Wrap your hands once (the backs of the hands touch) or twice (the left fingers come into the right palm).

- Inhale, lift bent elbows higher, but drop the shoulders.

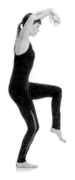
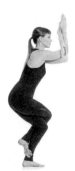
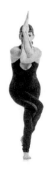

- Exhale, sit down deeper, and/or curl forward to hook the elbows in front of the top knee. Keep the feet charging down.

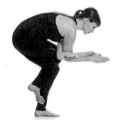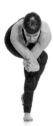

Breathe in Eagle Pose for 5 to 10 breaths; then unwind your feet to the floor, roll down, and repeat on the other side.

Ankle-to-Knee Chair Pose to Forward Fold

- Roll up, rooting the right foot and lifting the left knee.

- Cross your left ankle over your right knee.

- Open the bent knee toward the floor more, but lift your front top pelvis upward to clear the hip creases.

- Place your palms together in front of your chest. Inhale here.

- Exhale, sit down deeper, and lean forward to hook elbows in front of top shin. Keep the feet charging down.

- Activate your inner thighs into groins and out through the sitting bones, and draw your front lumbar spine in and up to stabilize from overcurving or tipping the pelvis too far forward.

- As an option, bend forward and touch the fingertips to the floor or a block. Straighten the standing leg more for a forward bend.

Breathe in the pose for 5 to 10 breaths; then unwind both feet to the floor, roll down, and repeat on the other side.

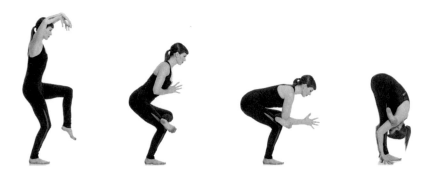

Dog Twist to Side Plank

Ground down all ten fingertips and the outer ring of your palm evenly to activate *hasta bandha* (hand arch support).

Begin in Downward-Facing Dog:

- ⟡ Lift your heels, bend your knees, and twist the knees to the right, heels to the left.

- ⟡ Press long through your right hand, and breathe to stretch all along your right waist.

- ⟡ Keep knees twisted to the right, and draw your lower belly in and up as you straighten your legs to come into Side Plank with one foot in front of the other on the floor.

- ⟡ Lift your right arm to the sky, if possible.

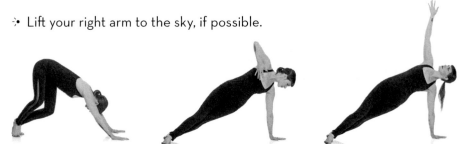

- ⟡ Beginners: to modify, bend your top leg, and plant the foot on the floor in front of you halfway up your mat.

Hold Side Plank for 1 to 5 breaths; then return to Downward-Facing Dog, and repeat Dog Twist to Side Plank on the left. Repeat Dog Twist to Side Plank on each side in a flow 3 to 5 times. Rest in Child's Pose.

When you finish, end with your Core Cooldown.

Namaste! Good job today.

FOOD

Balancing your diet is like Goldilocks's search for a comfy bed: not too hard, not too soft . . . but just right. Find what works to keep you in balance while still loving your meals. I want you to enjoy your food and eat just until you're satisfied (neither overstuffed nor joy-sucked and starving). Leave room to move, breathe, and be energetic, even as you digest.

You don't have to eat skinless chicken breasts and steamed broccoli in order to see real change in your body and vitality, either. When you eat 80 percent whole and healthy and 20 percent not so much, you will still end up eating well and craving less, because your body is getting much of the nutrition it needs. If you eat a diet devoid of vitamins and minerals, your body will, like the Cookie Monster, keep pushing you to shove more stuff in your mouth trying to seek its crucial building blocks.

Today, make the switch from being an imbalanced beast—to feeling your balanced best.

RECIPES

BREAKFAST: HOT LEMON DETOX

Lemons are one of nature's cool kids. They are one of the only anionic foods, which means that, like healing sea air and Himalayan salt lamps, they contain a negative ionic charge. Lemons are also chemically similar to your digestive juices and will cleanse your filter organs, like the kidneys and liver, kill bacteria, and help you digest your breakfast better.

My ayurvedic doctor suggests this as the only daily cleanse you need.

> half to whole lemon, squeezed
> 1 teaspoon honey (optional)
> 1 cup hot water

Boil the water in a teapot or an electric kettle (lifesaver!).

Pour the hot water into a teacup, and squeeze in lemon. Add honey if desired, and, after it cools just enough to drink, bottoms up! If the citrus is too much for your stomach, switch to an herbal detox tea or green tea instead.

SADIE'S MORNING SMOOTHIE: THE PB AND YAY!

Try my personal favorite and power up your potassium with a halved, frozen banana plus frozen peaches, peanut butter, yogurt, and add a spiral of honey on top. This will equal one big ol' glass of awesome.

I freeze peeled, halved bananas by the bunch to save time (and ice) in the morning.

SNACK: GREEK OUT

Take one organic Greek yogurt and turbo-charge its detox benefits by sprinkling with a few nuts or some ground flaxseed, and toss in some fresh or frozen fruit.

LUNCH: BEAUTIFUL BODY BOWL—GO QUIN-WILD

Make some quinoa, and as you cook it, toss in a wild thing, like dandelion greens or arugula. Squeeze some lemon over the whole thing to soften the greens more and make them more bio-available for your bod.

DINNER: GRILLED MAHIMAHI WITH APPLE-MANGO CHUTNEY

Serves 2

I got this crazy-good dish from my literary agent, Stephanie Tade, who somehow finds time to wow her dinner guests. The simple chutney takes a little time to cook, but it's so worth it. Make it in the morning or even the night before. You can refrigerate it and use the leftovers on everything from chicken to roast veggies for about a week.

FOR THE CHUTNEY

- 3 Granny Smith or other tart green apples, cored, peeled, and cut into half-inch dice
- 1 mango, peeled, seeded, and cut into chunks
- a good squirt of agave nectar
- 1/2 cup raisins (optional)
- 1 tablespoon red wine vinegar
- 1 tablespoon freshly squeezed lemon juice
- 1/2 yellow onion, diced
- pinch of salt
- pinch of red pepper flakes

FOR THE FISH MARINADE

- 1/2 cup orange juice
- 2 tablespoons soy sauce or wheat-free tamari
- spritz of lemon juice
- 1 tablespoon dark sesame oil or 1 teaspoon regular sesame oil mixed with 1 tablespoon canola oil
- 12 to 16 ounces mahimahi (or other grill-worthy, meaty fish like salmon, tuna, or swordfish)

Make the chutney

In a saucepan, mix all chutney ingredients. Cook on high for a few minutes until the mixture begins to bubble. Turn the heat down to medium-low, cover, and cook for about an hour, stirring occasionally. It should be pretty mushy. Remove pot from heat, let it cool, and pour the chutney into a covered container. Refrigerate until you're ready to use it.

Marinate the fish

In a nonreactive container large enough to hold the fish in one layer, whisk together all marinade ingredients. Place the fish in the marinade. Flip it a few times to coat. Cover the fish, put in the fridge, and let marinate for 20 minutes.

To grill your fish

Preheat the grill, and oil the grate. Take the fish out of marinade, and pat it dry. Sear the fish skin side down for 2 to 3 minutes; then flip and continue cooking until it's done. The rule is 10 minutes of cooking time for each inch of thickness.

To cook on the stove

Preheat an oiled grill pan until hot over medium-high heat. Follow the rest of the cooking instructions as for the grill.

Serve the fish topped with a generous spoonful of chutney with a side of quinoa casserole and/or steamed vegetable of choice. Drizzle the whole dish with lime juice and cracked pepper and sea salt to taste.

BEVERAGES

> Let's have a little fun: you have that 20 percent to cover.

FIZZY LEMONADE

I cannot live without this simple drink. Well, I could, but I don't want to. It's such a refreshing superdetox and has replaced all sugary soda pop for me.

> half to whole lemon
>
> 2 cups sparkling water
>
> 1 teaspoon agave nectar (optional)

Put a few ice cubes in a tall glass. Squeeze in the juice of half a lemon or more if you like living on the edge. Add a drizzle of agave if you want it sweetened. Fill the glass with sparkling water.

Wine 'n' Dine: White with Fish

It's a myth that white wine should always be paired with fish. Italians say the only rule is "wine with food"; however, I like a lighter glass with a more refined-tasting dinner.

My choice: A fruit-forward California or Oregon pinot noir, or a minerally French sauvignon blanc to balance the sweetness of the mango chutney.

ACTION: EIGHTY-TWENTY YOUR LIFE

During your day, do you spend as much time or more on your own nourishment, your own projects, and paying attention to yourself as you do for other people? Ninety-nine percent of the time, people's answer is no.

Working to make someone else's dreams happen to the point that you neglect your own, chronically disregarding your needs for the sake of anyone or anything else, just ain't cool. And more important, it doesn't work. Enabling people to avoid doing their own work and blocking them from learning their lessons is not helping them or you.

You can reorient your daily business so that it includes making your health and passion a priority and keeps you so full of energy that you have something more joyful to offer instead of resentment-tinged "should"-based actions. Today I want you to write down how you can shift a few things this week and begin to practice the following four things on most days.

My Fantastic Four Ways to Regain Your Balance Each Day

1. **Talk to the Hand:** Say "no" five times a day. Say it nicely . . . but say it. You'll see how many opportunities arise for you to do this when you put your mind to it.

2. **Work Out or In:** Start attending or go more frequently to an exercise program in your community. I'm partial to yoga, obviously, but signing up with a studio, gym, or running group, for example, infuses you with the energy of being with people and helps you commit to your health. If you can't find one you like, work "in"—online classes abound that you can do right in your living room.

3. **Eat a Power Breakfast:** Eat properly in the morning and you spark your metabolism and stabilize blood sugar, leaving you more energetic and balanced. Make your first meal rock and you won't be a hot mess by noon.

4. **Assume the Best:** If you're stressing about a situation, see what happens if, instead of bracing for the worst, you decide to trust the process, release the outcome, and get back to doing things that keep you chillaxed and on your own best path.

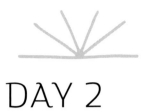

DAY 2

THEME: Get Your Ass in Gear

When I first decided to move from a joy-sucking corporate cubicle job into something I loved that was aligned with me—heart and soul—I heard two words a lot from those around me: "You can't..." For instance:

"You can't make money in yoga."

"You can't excel in the wellness field—there's too much competition."

"You can't be stable in that career—are you crazy? What about your 401(k)?"

I had two words to say back to that kind of negativity: "Watch me."

So years later—with a more than comfortable income, bestselling DVDs, a TV show, this book with my dream publisher, and a world-traveling, love- and magic-filled life sharing the things I'm most passionate about—when I am asked the question "How did you get this life?" my answer is always the same: "I didn't follow my dreams, or wait for them...I *made* them happen."

The difference between people who create miracle transformations in their lives, who live their dreams out loud instead of only in their mind, and those who don't comes down to this: those who were not satisfied with their current situations, then changed them for the better, all did one thing... *they did something about it.*

When I brought my completed manuscript for my first book, *Road Trip Guide to the Soul,* to my first literary agent, she said something that struck me: "Sadie, there are so many people out there who could write a book, and should write a book, but never will. Congratulations, you're now part of the vast minority who actually wrote one."

I have two books now—because I lived them, and then I wrote them.

I hear frustrated clients lament over and over again that they would get to their dreams, *if only*. If only the stars would align, and somehow they would find the time to do something for themselves within all the demands of the kids, the relationship, the job, the bills, the commitments they have made.

If only the money would come. If only they were hotter. If only they could find time for the vacation. If only they were clearer about how to begin. If only they were sure they were good enough or confident enough.

If only.

Well, guess what? *If only* never comes. That's because all of these things are an outcome of taking actions that are aligned with your truth. You create confidence by doing your own work and seeing it work out on your behalf.

Manifesting your dreams is like breaking in new cowgirl boots; you just have to start with what you got, push on in there, and stretch yourself out some space until they fit perfectly.

If you feel frustrated, stuck, and unsure how to get yourself from here to there, the one thing that you definitely should do first is . . . anything.

That is, anything that moves you in the direction of your best body, mind, heart, and self-expression, instead of away from it. In every moment, there are a million places to start. Pick one. Begin to live as you want to become, right now. To do this, switch your *if onlys* to *even if*.

You can improve your life on every level, right now, even if you only have five minutes. Even if you have one dollar to your name. Even if you're busy, stressed, and tired. Even if. People with more problems than you have done it—and you can, too.

When you decide to make it happen, you will begin to see, and then use, every possible opportunity to chip away at that big concrete block that seems to be standing in the way of freedom, empowerment, health, wealth, and fitness. You'll find that rock will soon be nothing but a pile of dust for all your doubts to eat as you speed onward. So, let's get your ass in gear . . . and onto the mat.

YOGA

Today's sequence will help you get the most bang from your yoga buck. If you're going to take actions, I want them to move you forward in the most efficient way. Because you are working every transition and pose more than usual, you really are getting the benefits of two poses every time you do one. This means that if you replace 20 minutes of watching TV or surfing the web with 20 minutes of this yoga, it's like doing 40 minutes of many other styles and exercises. You will see results faster for the same time you spend on your mat. Let's do this. Not half-asana'd . . . but full on.

Begin with 3 to 5 rounds of your Core Warm-Up.

Temple Arch/Curl to Twisted Temple

Work your whole lower body as you resist and release your leg, shoulder, lower back, and chest muscles for a sweet stretch. The spinal movement helps you release stored energy and refocus your best intentions.

- Come to stand at the front of your mat, and then step your feet really wide—off your mat.

- Turn your toes out to face the same way as your knees as you bend your legs, and reach down to plant your fingertips on the mat or two blocks.

- Beginners: If you can't reach this low, place your hands or forearms on your thighs instead.

- Open your knees wider to stretch the inner thighs and groin.

- Inhale, and arch your back. As you do, bend your knees even more.

- Exhale, round your back, and engage your front spine and lower belly in and up.

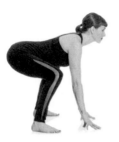 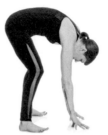

- Repeat the arch/curl for about 1 minute or longer. Pause and take multiple breaths at any point in the pose that you feel needs more opening.

- When you're finished, press your right foot and hand into the floor or block, and reach your left arm up. Bend the elbow, and flip your palm up to thread the back of your hand onto your back or even into the right hip crease for a half-bound arm position.

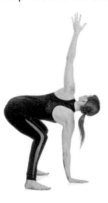

- Inhale, ground through your feet, and wave length through your spine.

- Exhale, and spin your chest and left shoulder toward the sky.

- Look down at the floor to stretch the neck and top shoulder.

- Straighten your legs a little more if possible, and play the edge of your stretch.

- Take 5 breaths here; then release and repeat the sequence from Temple Arch/Curl and Twisted Temple on the right side.

- End in a wide forward bend, folding to center for 5 breaths.

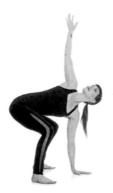
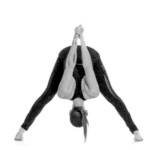

Fierce Chair Pose Sequence

This sequence amps up your fierceness, releases emotional blocks, and gives a blissful release through the whole Core Strength Muscle Meridian and outer body.

- Step both feet to the front of your mat and widen them about hip-distance.

- Roll down over bent legs, and "rag-doll" your body into a gentle forward bend.

- Bend your knees a lot so that your belly is on your thighs.

- Root your feet, and lift the toes.

- Exhale, and roll up over your bent legs. Front pelvis lifts, and inhale as arms unroll to the sky.

- Inhale, prepare.

- Exhale, stick your tongue out (Lion's Roar), and say "Ahhhhh!" Go wild. Wake the neighbors. As you roar, bend over, swing Fists of Fire past your hips, and open your hands behind you in a "throw-it-away" motion.

- Inhale, and roll back up into Fierce Chair Pose, so-named because of your fiery intention to let go of any obstacles to your freedom.

- Play with your Fierce Chair, floating arms up on the inhale, and on the exhales doing Fists of Fire into Lion's Roar.

Repeat the sequence 5 to 10 times.

- On your last exhale, interlace your fingers behind your back.

- Inhale, press feet down, lift the pelvis up, and cascade your spine down over your strong legs.

- Exhale; end in a clasped-hand Forward Fold.

- Take 5 breaths here; then release hands to shins or floor into Forward Fold for another 5 breaths.

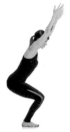 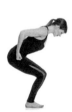 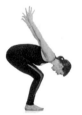 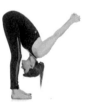

Return to the beginning of the sequence, and repeat all the way through on the opposite side.

When you finish, end with your Core Cooldown.

Namaste! Good job today.

FOOD

I know you're busy. I'm busy, too. When I look at a recipe book and think about organizing myself, not to mention the multiple ingredients needed to cook even one meal, my...brain...explodes. Yet I have found ways to make supernutritious meals with minimal effort—and they taste great!

Today I want you to see how easy it can be to cook simply and more healthfully—in less time—so I've designed all the recipes to be fast, to be filling, and to build you up with more iron and protein to conquer all your Yoga Body tasks today.

RECIPES

BREAKFAST: IRON(WO)MAN FRICKTTATA

Today, multitask your meal. Add some spinach to your frittata; then have a small glass of OJ or half a grapefruit—the citrus makes the iron in the spinach more available to your body.

LUNCH: POWER LUNCH SMOOTHIE

Blend your smoothie today with a high-pro glow—add another tablespoon of almond or cashew butter, some Greek yogurt, or a scoop of protein powder to power you through the busy day!

DINNER: SADIE'S SKILLET SALAD

Tonight, mix in some spinach, sliced garlic, cherry tomatoes, cashews, and a splash of balsamic vinegar. Add dried cranberries or mandarin orange slices for a sweet surprise.

SNACKS: STOCK YOUR BAR

It's fine to grab a snack bar; just make sure it's one of the more balanced brands that don't spike your blood sugar and aren't superprocessed. You want to look for a smaller gap between protein grams and carbs, and also some healthy fats. A few of my faves are

P.S.: If you want to be a superwoman and also save money, make your own bars. Check out my gluten-free, protein-packed Rock-n-Rolled Oats and Quinoa Energy Bar recipe, which follows.

- *Luna Bar:* great blend of the Big 3: protein, whole carbs, healthy fat. Sweeter than most for a feeling of indulgence. I love their Nutz Over Chocolate and Chai flavors.

- *Kind:* Chock-full o' nuts and real fruit, these bars are naturally balanced and widely available.

- *Yoga Earth:* Formulated by scientists and yogis to be awesome, they even have a chocolate-covered quinoa-based line of bars (Keen Wah Decadence).

- *Pure:* Lower in protein but fully organic and made with all raw fruit and nut ingredients for a satisfying snack.

ROCK-N-ROLLED OATS AND QUINOA ENERGY BAR

Makes 8 to 12 bars

2 cups organic quick-cooking rolled oats

1/2 cup quinoa, cooked

1/2 cup organic protein powder (optional—between the quinoa and nuts, you'll be fine for protein)

1/4 cup ground flaxseed or chia seeds or a combination

1 teaspoon baking soda

1/2 teaspoon sea salt

1 cup raw almonds

1/2 cup dried fruit of choice (dates, cherries, cranberries all work well alone or in combination)

1/2 cup shredded coconut

1/2 cup buckwheat flour

1 cup water

1 teaspoon cinnamon

1/4 cup honey

1/4 cup olive oil (or replace with half a mashed banana)

2 teaspoons organic vanilla extract

Preheat the oven to 350°F. Grease a 9 x 13-inch pan with a little organic butter or organic canola spray. Combine everything in a large bowl. Stir until flour is mixed evenly throughout. Spoon mixture into pan; use your fingers to press and fit to the edges.

Bake for 20 minutes. Let cool on the stovetop for 20 minutes. Cut into bars and serve. Store extras in an airtight dish in the fridge or freeze, tightly wrapped.

Bars last a week without freezing.

DESSERT: FRUIT SUNDAE

Since your dinner is so low-cal, add something to seal the deal: top a dollop of coconut ice cream with some of your smoothie frozen fruit, or puree your own really quicky. Frozen-raspberry-and-peach mixes are my jam.

BEVERAGES: BODACIOUS BERRY TEA INFUSION

This is a great way to work more healing properties of tea into your diet. Keep a jar of this in the fridge, and enjoy all day long. Makes a great vodka cocktail base too . . . just sayin'.

5 tea bags of hibiscus or other berry-based tea

10 cups filtered water

1 lime, sliced, plus more for garnish

1 lemon, sliced

1 cup frozen berries of choice

Brew tea in a teapot or pan on the stove. Pour into a heat-safe pitcher. Add the fruit, and cool in the fridge for 30 minutes.

In a tall glass, pour over ice, garnish with one lime slice, and serve.

ACTION: THE 5-MINUTE REVOLUTION

When it comes to making changes, many people have an all-or-nothing approach: "If I don't have a thousand dollars in the bank, I can't take a vacation." Well, welcome to shooting yourself in the foot. Hurts, doesn't it?

This black-and-white mentality leads to waiting forever to be happy, rested, sane, and creative, instead of doing whatever you can right now to move toward your dreams, *even as you live them*—which is a whole lot more satisfying. When you do nothing, you create nothing. For example, let's say your expertise is in using social media to sell more effectively. You could write out "The Top 10 Ways to Make Money Online."

Have it edited and designed, and stick some pretty pictures in there from a free photo site. Lock it into a PDF, and send an e-mail blast, post about it on Facebook, create a landing page, sell it—hey, you're the social media guru.

What more could you do from here? Lots. Because, ultimately, the dedicated work you do toward your dream builds on itself and will keep expanding—if you *just do it* . . . and to do that, you must begin. So what will you do today, even if you only have 5 minutes, to take that next step? Your dream is waiting . . . now go get it.

Today, begin to take baby bites out of your larger goals. Use your imagination, too, but here are a few things you could do in a few moments to move yourself in your new, empowering direction.

5-Minute Revolutions

❖ **Go Eco-chic**: Make your coffee and snacks at home, and bring your own reuseable water bottle. Put the $5 to $15 you would have spent each day on these incidentals into a piggy bank "vacation fund" or whatever you want to save for. It adds up faster than you might imagine, even if you don't do it every day.

❖ **Barter Blitz**: Write an e-mail to one person you want to trade or partner with in some way to help you move forward. Maybe you are an accountant and you also want to do yoga. Some teacher or studio in town is going to guest you into their classes in exchange for a tax return. Get creative—what do you need, and what do you have to offer? I do this all the time and get so much done without spending money.

❖ **Multitasker Workout**: Do 5 minutes of exercise while watching TV in front of the couch instead of sitting on it. That's 35 minutes of benefits you weren't getting each week—but you are now.

❖ **Minimeditation**: Sit, breathe, and reflect on your present moment. Five minutes—heck, 5 breaths—gives you a clarity and calm that is so much more valuable than 5 minutes of reading PerezHilton.com (but, OK, maybe not as fun).

Brainstorm on it, and write down a few of your own 5-Minute Revolutions for this week. Add at least one for today. Then . . . just do it.

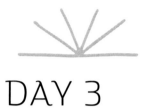

DAY 3

THEME: Kicking Logs

At a yoga and empowerment training in Asheville, North Carolina, I was leading a discussion about how to make the personal changes you desire when other people in your life seem to be resistant to supporting healthy shifts in you, or themselves.

One woman described how frustrated she was becoming with her husband of twenty-plus years. The adventurous guy who originally attracted her is now more likely to be found parked in the La-Z-Boy, third beer in hand, than out and about with her.

Recently, she managed to drag him, reluctantly, along on a hike. While they were up on the trail, she tripped and kicked over a log. Under the log was a roiling mass of bugs that scattered to find new cover. At first, she thought, "Oooh! I'm so sorry!" Then she paused, seeing things in a new light: "Why am I sorry? What if I just took a big weight off of those bugs' backs and gave them a whole bunch of new possibilities!" She walked on, thinking, "You're welcome, guys!" All the other class participants roared with laughter, because they could relate to those bugs. People do the same old things under the same old log, day in and day out, waiting for things to move or for someone else to come along and kick it off. And when that happens, boy, is it hard for many people to tear themselves away from the faux-comfort of living under the compression they are accustomed to.

Maybe you won't like the sudden feeling of expansion, lightness, and energy that comes when the weight of that log is gone. You're so exposed, unsure and blinking in the light.

So then what? Do you scramble back under that familiar place? Or do you go your own way, seek another path, and create a home that's more your style?

And, dear reader, please don't spend another minute trying to shove off *other* people's logs. It's none of your business. Swing your foot back, and take aim for the only log you need to let fly: your own. Whether or not those around you choose to come on your grand adventures is also not your concern. They will or they won't, and later you can think about what you need to do to respect their truth but still rock yours. Today, you will begin to lose some excess weight, on any level you feel necessary, and lighten up. Take this opportunity to start investigating and inhabiting your possibilities, and begin to reclaim your right to live fully in the sun . . . because honey, you deserve it.

YOGA

In yoga, we call log-kicking *Tapas*, or getting radically present, shaking things up, then delivering a kung-fu roundhouse kick to any obstacles in front of your inherent freedom and joy. It's the first, foundational step toward any process of transformation.

I often speak about the weight-loss benefits of my style of yoga, but I don't promote becoming a skinny girl. Skinnier is not always better. Eating is fun, and I want you to be fit and strong, not scrawny and dry as beef jerky.

I want us all to reclaim the notion of "losing weight" as a more holistic process of shedding anything that is an obstacle to your health and Core Strength. If you're a juicy, curvy yogi, and you are healthy and empowered, that's brilliant. If you're naturally thin and lean at your set point, then that's where you want to be.

If you, however, have physical pounds that need to go so that you can avoid obesity-related disease, then I'd say you're in the right place, as well. Hanging on to too thin or too fat for your healthy type is another log that needs kickin'.

Weight is not just physical either. If you have emotional or mental baggage you have carried with you into this moment, then I encourage you to retain the lesson but thank your teachers—then leave the luggage they handed to you back at their feet and walk on. Today's practice will help you drop any excess heaviness like a hot potato—and move forward with a happy spring in your step.

Begin with 3 to 5 rounds of your Core Warm-Up.

Kicking Logs Flow

Kick of Fire: This will activate your solar plexus, the seat of willpower, and strengthen your body, along with the fierce resolve to make real changes in your life.

- ❂ Begin in Downward-Facing Dog.

- ❂ Inhale as your right foot lifts. Exhale through Core Plank to step your right foot to right thumb.

- ❂ Come into High Lunge.

- ❂ Inhale, and lean torso forward. Reach your arms up by your ears.

- ❂ Step your back foot forward a little for balance.

- ❂ Exhale, and all at once pull Fists of Fire down to your hips, and bend right knee up into your chest as you stand. Draw your lower belly in and up as you kick your right leg forward through a strong heel. Say "Ha!"

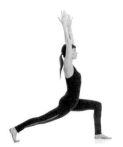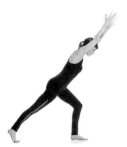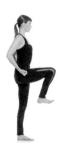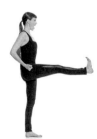

Repeat Kick of Fire 5 times. Return to High Lunge and take a Vinyasa flow to Downward-Facing Dog. Repeat Kick of Fire on the left 5 times. Repeat the whole sequence 3 times on each leg. On your last round, proceed to Lakshmi Kick.

Kick of Fire to Lakshmi Kick: The goddess Lakshmi is the symbol of prosperity and beauty—two things you'll get from this cleansing inversion, which also lightens your emotional load.

❖ From your last Kick of Fire stance on your right standing leg, bend both knees and fold forward to plant your fingertips wide on the floor or blocks. Your left foot stays planted. Your right knee draws into your chest.

❖ Inhale, prepare.

❖ Exhale, kick your right leg out behind you through a strong heel as high as you can, and say "Ha!" as loud as you want.

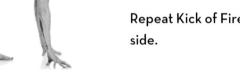

❖ Inhale, and bend both knees in again.

Repeat Lakshmi Kick 5 times or more. Then

❖ Bend your knees, roll up, and stretch arms overhead into Mountain Pose.

❖ Exhale, fold forward, and step or hop back to Downward-Facing Dog.

Repeat Kick of Fire to Lakshmi Kick on the other side.

When you finish, end with your Core Cooldown.

Namaste! Good job today.

FOOD

Last night I joined my friend Nikki at his apartment for dinner. Nikki is Indian and steeped in the ayurvedic tradition, an ancient healing system. He's also an amazing cook. I had such a fantastic dinner with Nikki that I asked him to create a meal plan for you today based on filling up without feeling heavy.

When it comes to eating any meal, the first priority is to eat mindfully and slowly, and to savor it. It takes 20 minutes for your brain to signal your stomach that you've had enough food, and you don't want to Hoover down your food so fast that you miss the moment that you start to become satisfied, not stuffed. Filled to the gills is yet another log we get to kick away today.

RECIPES

BREAKFAST: KICKING CLOGS JUICE

Morning is the perfect time to flush any toxic stuff clogging your pipes, so try adding in this Roto-Rooter combination of blood and filter-organ cleaners plus fiber—that also tastes kickin'.

- 2 apples, halved
- half a lemon, squeezed
- 4 packed cups kale or spinach, de-stemmed
- 2¾-inch cube peeled fresh ginger

SNACK: GUAC AND AWE

Serves 2

FYI: You can make a version of this really fast by mashing avocados, organic salsa, lime juice (or a little lemon if you don't have lime), and sea salt. But if you want to go the whole nine (minutes) . . . do this:

You *must* know about lentil chips. They're high in protein and taste so good. Pair a few with Nikki's handmade guacamole and some salsa for a perfect, lightly filling snack.

2 ripe avocados, slightly mushy to the touch

½ red onion, minced

1 tablespoon serrano chiles or jalapeño peppers, stems and seeds removed, minced

2 tablespoons cilantro leaves and tender stems, finely chopped

1 tablespoon fresh lime or lemon juice

½ teaspoon sea salt

black pepper to taste

½ ripe tomato, seeds and pulp removed, chopped

Cut the avocados in half. Remove the pits, and scoop out the rest into a bowl. Using a fork, roughly mash the avocado. Add other ingredients except tomato, and mash more to desired consistency.

Press plastic wrap directly onto the surface of the guacamole to prevent it from turning an unappetizing brown. Refrigerate until ready to serve; then add the tomato and mix together. Garnish with a few lentil chips, and serve with a bowl of chips on the side.

LUNCH: SWEET AND SAVORY SALAD

Add ¼ cup of cheese to your salad and a sprinkle of nuts to ground it, so it's light but not airy-fairy. I love goat cheese and walnuts sautéed in a little balsamic vinegar, honey, and black pepper in a pan.

DINNER: THE MONSTER MASH

Serves 2—or make 4 to store!

This dish is so massively good for you, it's a nutritional wild thing.

BOOST THE FLAVOR: A few dashes of curry powder (to taste) are great with this dish. Otherwise, you could add 2-cloves of garlic, chopped, or ½-cup coconut milk or chili powder (a few dashes, to taste).

1 tablespoon olive oil

6 ounces protein of choice, chopped (Nikki used tofu)

¼ cup cashews

2 tomatoes, chopped

1 green chile, de-seeded and finely chopped

½ cup green peas or edamame, fresh or frozen

salt and pepper to taste

In a medium-hot pan, heat olive oil, and sauté all ingredients until lightly browned and your protein of choice is cooked through. Add seasonings to taste as you cook.

Serve your Monster Mash on top of brown rice or quinoa, or stir it all together!

BEVERAGES: MATCHA GREEN TEA LATTE

Nikki wants me to turn you on to matcha. Matcha is a powdered green tea that has a nice, sustainable energy boost; doesn't make you as jittery or as likely to crash as coffee; and tastes more mellow than regular green tea leaves. Here's the way I love it.

matcha green tea powder (regular green tea will also do, if you can't find matcha)

1 cup plain unsweetened almond milk

agave nectar, honey, or vanilla extract to taste

Hot:

Sift 1 teaspoon matcha powder into a cup. Add 1/4 cup hot water, and stir until the mix becomes a smooth paste.

Heat the almond milk in a pan, and whisk until foamy. (I have a battery-operated frothing wand.) Stir agave nectar, honey, or vanilla into the milk if desired. Pour the milk mixture into the matcha paste, and whisk to blend. Pour into a cup and scoop any foam on top.

Sprinkle with a pinch of matcha dust or cocoa powder.

Iced:

Put some ice into a tall glass; then fill half the glass with cold almond milk and the rest with brewed matcha.

Sprinkle with a pinch of matcha dust or cocoa powder.

ACTION: THREE WAYS TO KICK A LOG

Look around yourself. Are there habits, beliefs, actions, or agreements that are smashing you like a little bug down in the muck?

If so, what could you do, right now, to move that log just a little—and, as the Band sings, "Take a load off?" Here are some of my favorite ways to do just that. You can create your own, write a list, and post it where you'll see it every day. When you get that log to move in a new empowering direction, write "KICKED!" after it. So satisfying.

Kick a Habit: What habitual actions have you been taking that are keeping you stuck or unhealthy in some way? How can you shift things, immediately? I used to drink loads of diet soda, aka fizzy neurotoxin. I switched it to soda water with agave and lemon, and my near-daily headaches and nerve tingling went away. **_KICKED!_**

Kick a Thought: You, like everyone except perhaps for the Dalai Lama, hold some beliefs about yourself and the world that can keep you in a rut of negativity and limitation. Question and confront them. I used to be certain that I had a terrible memory for names, so I wouldn't even try to remember those of my students. I called longtime students "Hey, Girlfriend" for years. Then I started to pay more attention and make it a higher priority to learn them, and—surprise! I could. **_KICKED!_**

Kick-Start a Project: Write down three ways you can get a passion project party started. At one point, I had this book to write, yet life still goes on, and it's easy to say yes to fun social engagements. So I placed a Monday through Friday moratorium on anything not directly book-related until it was done. Saturday and Sunday were fair game, though. You're reading this book, so you know that I **_KICKED!_**

Now you.

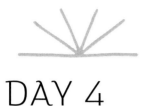

DAY 4

THEME: Become the Master

I was walking home from dinner at about 9:30 p.m., using a route I've taken a hundred times before. People were out and about, coming back from dinner.

I was texting a friend and didn't notice the young man running up behind me until I felt a strong yank on my purse. My first thought was that my dinner date had snuck up on me to walk me home and was trying to surprise me. Then the yank became a crazy-hard pull, and my purse strap broke off.

I reflexively grabbed my purse, and my cell phone clattered to the ground in front of me. The mugger ran a few paces down the street, realized he didn't have my purse, then turned back around, as if undecided whether he should get the hell out of Dodge or come back for a second try.

We looked at each other and in that moment, I had to think fast. I would have been happy to give him what he wanted, but I pondered what I could do to make him leave without taking my valuables, and not hurt me. That would be the best outcome for all involved, even for him, because then he wouldn't be a thief.

Luckily, my twenty-year yoga practice has given me some skills I didn't know would apply to a street mugging: the ability to slow down, breathe, and think more clearly—and take decisive action from this space rather freaking out. So, when my attacker took a couple of tentative steps toward me, I lunged for my iPhone, pointed it at him, and pretended to take a picture. Now hyperaware, I turned and did the same to his friend, who was coming down the other side of the street toward me.

I yelled, "I have both of your faces on camera, and I just texted them to my friend who's a police officer. He's on his way. You better run before they get here, or you're going to jail! Even if you take this phone right now or hurt me, the police still have your photos."

The two guys looked at each other, confused, then back at me. I yelled louder, "RUN!"

They turned and sprinted around the corner.

When I got to my apartment, I started shaking and did a few Sun Salutations to calm myself down. Assessing the damage, I had a broken purse and my arm was black-and-blue. It could have been much, much worse.

Part of the art of attention is drawing clear boundaries around your own health and safety, and the right to move through your days as a master, not a victim.

There's a Zen saying, *Trust everyone . . . but lock your doors at night.* The Victim sees everything as something being done *to him* (or her). And so it is.

The Master views all experiences as lessons happening *for him* (or her)—for his or her continued growth, strengthening, and wisdom. And so it is. Which you choose is up to you. You can begin to use each situation that you run into (or that runs into you, as the case may be) to more stubbornly become a Mindful Warrior.

If those dudes had been carrying guns, I would not have made the same choice. "Here's my purse, kind sirs" might have been the best way, and then I could take the photos so that they didn't think they could get away with murder.

Above all, be vigilant and know that in any relationship with another person, from the ones closest to you to the total strangers who appear in your life unexpectedly, you can be the Master or the Victim. The choice is yours. It's all how you decide to see it and move forward from there.

YOGA

In yoga, we see drawing a masterful boundary as the spiritual "no way," a crucial counterbalance to your "yes, totally." The practice of Core Strength living is to know what to choose but also what *not* to choose. And remember: if it's not a big loud *yes* in your heart, it's a *no*. When your choices are put into service of your right to stay full, energetic, effective, and accomplishing your soul projects, you will invite in a rush of new energy instead of draining it out for everyone else's benefit.

Today, as you immerse in Warrior I and the Temple Stance, be aware of your tendencies to give out too much energy or movement in a place that isn't as necessary, such as gripping too hard or going so deep that you lose your foundational grounding and core alignment. Back off, soften, or hug in that misdirected energy, and get back to mastering your pose, not becoming a victim of it.

Begin with 3 to 5 rounds of your Core Warm-Up.

Bridge between poses or flows with a Vinyasa flow sequence whenever you wish.

Inner Warrior/Temple Flow

Warrior I and Temple Stance are linked together for whole-body toning, grounding, and energy. Warrior poses give you the stamina to break through resistance and fly higher.

Warrior I: Come into Downward-Facing Dog.

◌ Inhale, and lift your left leg into Dog Split.

◌ Exhale through Core Plank to step left foot to left thumb.

◌ Inhale, and wave your spine long.

◌ Exhale and at the same time ground your back foot down naturally (toes will face semiforward at about 45 degrees) as you root the feet, lift your front pelvis, and begin to roll up.

- Inhale, unfurl the arms overhead, chest faces forward. This is Warrior I.

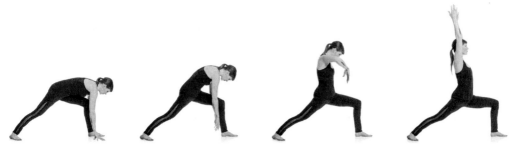

Your kneecap and toes should always face the same direction. It's easy to twist the back knee in this pose by trying to square the hips forward. Forget that—instead, let your hips face diagonally toward the upper left corner of your mat. Twist forward only from the chest and higher. Make this an empowering core strength pose, too.

- Take 5 breaths here. Now fly into Fierce Temple.

Fierce Temple

- Lean your whole torso forward, and fly your arms back behind you like Superman for Flying Warrior I.

- Inhale, prepare.

- Exhale, sweep your left arm down and forward, and then follow it up and open it back behind you as you open the back hip and foot.

- Position both feet open in the same direction as your knees, and bend both knees wide.

- In Temple, bend your right elbow over your left, and wrap forearms and hands if possible.

- Inhale, arch your spine, and lift elbows up.

- Exhale, stick your tongue out, and say "Haaaaah" and round forward. This stimulates your solar plexus, seat of willpower.

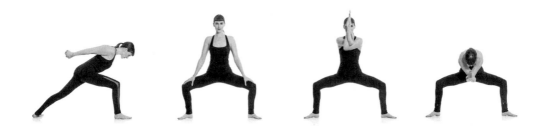

Repeat Fierce Temple 5 to 10 times. Then turn front toes forward, back heel lifts into a high lunge position. Plant your hands at the front of your mat, and return to Downward-Facing Dog. Repeat flow from Warrior I on the other side. Repeat the whole flow 1 to 3 times on each side.

FOOD

I used to be a victim of my cravings. I could be aiming to eat less sugar, but one inquiry of "you want this box of chocolates, Sadie?" would result in a freakishly quick: "Hells to the yeah!" This kind of self-placating behavior might be momentarily delicious but can wreck your long-term ability to reach your more important goals.

One day my friend looked at my chocolate-stained mouth and said, "You really aren't that strong, willpower-wise, are you?" I realized I wasn't fully living up to my potential, and it wasn't cute that I didn't trust myself not to self-sabotage.

If you're trying to switch to a healthier way of approaching food, seesawing hunger hormones can weaken your best intentions and stop you dead in your tracks. Cravings can be the result of eating nonnutritious and processed foods, not eating enough, or only eating sugar or other simple carbs. Other factors are your body's reactions to hormonal fluctuations, using food as an emotional coping mechanism, and a blood-sugar imbalance.

If you know how and when your body is likely to become reactive, you can say no to those behaviors and yes to actions that preempt blood sugar or mood swings and keep yourself on a more even keel. Today's menu gives your body the proper nutrition and hydration it's often craving when it cries out for more food, so you can stay in mastery of your diet.

RECIPES

BREAKFAST: QUINOA CEREAL

Everything that gives you something, like sudden energy, will balance the equation by taking something away later. Grab a cup of sugary coffee or carb-laden food in the morning and you're likely to crash and dash—straight to more quick fixes that aren't good for you. Instead, try a protein-rich first meal that will give you long-lasting fuel to keep you on top of your game all day long.

¼ cup quinoa

½ cup filtered water

pinch of sea salt

¼ cup fresh or dried fruit

¼ cup nuts

1 tablespoon ground flaxseeds or chia seeds

½ cup milk (my pick: unsweetened vanilla almond milk)

2 teaspoons agave nectar or honey

Make quinoa with water and salt in a rice cooker or pan. When done, transfer to a cereal bowl, and top with the fruit, nuts, and seeds; then pour milk over all. Drizzle with agave nectar or honey and serve.

SNACKS: NEWTON'S NOSH

Slice an apple, and then to ground the carbs and your blood sugar, spread some nut butter on each slice. Sunflower butter is incredible here. Dust lightly with cinnamon and you're good to go.

LUNCH: BLT SALAD

This is a healthy alternative to the greasy-spoon BLT, and it's just as delicious. More so, actually, because it's as good for you as it tastes.

2 cups salad greens

1 cup chopped ripe tomato

1/2 ripe avocado, chopped

1/4 red onion, sliced paper-thin

1 tablespoon olive oil or Creamy Garlic Dressing (see recipe on page 17)

sea salt, cracked pepper to taste

1 strip of organic turkey or veggie bacon, cooked and cooled

In a salad bowl, mix all the ingredients except the bacon. Toss the salad to coat with dressing, and season with sea salt and cracked pepper to taste. Garnish with crumbled bacon and serve.

DINNER: QUICK TOMATO-CARROT-BASIL SOUP

Serves 2

Yes, it's soooo Julia Child–chic to simmer homemade soup for hours on the stove; however, when you don't have time for that, try the next best thing: a fresh, tasty soup that takes about 15 minutes from fridge to table.

2 cups organic veggie stock

1 cup chopped baby carrots

2 tomatoes, diced

1 to 2 stalks celery, chopped

1/4 red onion, diced

1 clove garlic, crushed (optional, unless you're me; then it's nonnegotiable)

1 teaspoon finely chopped fresh basil or 1/2 teaspoon dried basil

dash of sea salt and cracked pepper

NOTE: Refrigerating tomatoes depletes their flavor, so keep them on the counter.

Put all the ingredients into a blender, and blend on High to your preferred consistency. Put in a pot, heat it, and eat it. Stir in 1/2 cup cooked brown rice or quinoa for an even heartier meal. Or eat it with some of your lentil chips. Garnish with a sprig of basil, crumbled turkey bacon, and/or some goat cheese if desired. You can even eat this at room temperature or chilled for a gazpacho-style dish.

DESSERT: RAW MEXICAN CHOCOLATE MACAROONS

Makes 10 macaroons or more, depending on how you roll

I found this gem on my travels through Mexico. It's one of my supremely popular recipes (with me as much as my dinner guests) and tastes far more decadent than it is. The secret is the three Cs: cocoa, cinnamon, and cayenne. Caliente!

I serve these with pretty little macchiatos: decaf or regular espressos topped with a dollop of steamed coconut milk.

1¼ cups shredded sweetened or unsweetened coconut	2 tablespoons sweetener, like maple syrup, honey, or agave nectar
¼ cup cold-pressed extra-virgin coconut oil	½ teaspoon vanilla extract
	a few shakes of cinnamon powder
5 tablespoons cocoa powder	sprinkle of cayenne pepper

Put all ingredients into a blender. Scrape and blend until thoroughly mixed.

Roll the mix into small balls you could eat in a few bites. Place in a nonstick dish or on waxed paper on a cooking tray in the fridge. After about 10 minutes, the macaroons should be set. Serve on a pretty white plate sprinkled with extra cocoa, cayenne, and cinnamon.

BEVERAGE: CHAI LATTE

I drink a chai latte nearly every morning with breakfast, unless I'm in Mexico, in which case, I drink a mango margarita. Kidding . . . kind of.

Chai is made with black tea and spices. It's delicious and warming, and it wakes you up without the sharp jolt of coffee. I've refined it from the sugary concoction I used to order at my local coffee shop. Now I make it at home. I often have a decaf version of chai for dessert. This is also delicious iced.

1 cup milk or milk alternative	agave nectar or honey to taste
1 to 2 chai tea bags	cinnamon, for garnish
1 cup hot water	

Heat the milk in a pan on medium-low on the stove. Stir milk often until warm. Put 1 to 2 chai tea bags in a teacup and fill three-quarters to the top with boiling water. Let steep for 3 minutes, remove the bags, and add a squeeze of agave or honey and stir. Fill the rest of the cup with milk. Stir. Garnish with cinnamon and serve.

ACTION: PAY ATTENTION MEDITATION

Today I'm asking you to purchase some colorful sticky notes and a pen with an ink color that also appeals to you (I'm partial to silver). Write "ATTENTION" on each sticky note. Put them in the places where you tend to go the most and want a reminder to check in with yourself and be high-quality present:

- on the dash of your car

- by your computer screen

- inside the fridge

- on the bathroom mirror

- next to your TV

- inside your significant other's brain (heheh!)

When you see one of the notes, do one of the following:

- Breathe deeper.

- Ask "Is the action I'm taking/about to take going to represent and serve me best?" (before sending a bitchy e-mail, for example).

- Get up, stretch, and move around.

- Do something that will help you realize your dreams.

- Have a healthy meal or beverage. Yes, wine counts.

- Close your eyes, and let your thoughts play elsewhere while your mind clears.

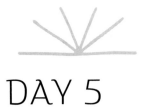

DAY 5

THEME: Deny Drama

As I write this, I'm sitting at a beach bar in Turks and Caicos, with a glass of cold pinot grigio in one hand, pen in the other. I'm on a balcony facing the ocean and looking at what just might go down in my record books as one of the most beautiful sunsets ever. The only thing marring my moment of Zen is the woman at the next table talking whiny-loud to her friend: "Oh. My. Gawd. This has been the *worst* day, like, *ever*! I lost my keys in the morning and totally freaked out, like, for *hours*. I couldn't even go to the beach. I was like, Ben's going to kill me, they had our apartment keys on them! And then I was too stressed to even enjoy my lunch!" (Insert more of the same, for twenty straight minutes.)

I want to get in her face and tell her to zip it so that everyone could enjoy in peace the amazing watercolor Mother Nature is painting, fleetingly, just for us. But what I do instead is take a deep breath, drop my resistance to reality, and redirect it toward the view, my wine, and you, dear reader.

It's so easy to become a drama junkie, addicted to the rush of adrenaline. The heightened awareness that comes with that rush is the opposite of the kind you get during meditation. It's your lizardy animal brain going into overdrive until the feeling of world domination passes and your world comes crashing down on you like a poorly constructed tent in the rain. No thanks.

I prefer my intensity to come with a side of healing, joy, and the freedom to do my own best work that day.

When I first tried to deny drama, it was hard to disengage. I kept returning for the toxic juice, the sick, hopeful feeling that I could make a difference by entangling myself in power struggles. It was about as effective as beating my head against a brick wall. Then I realized: drama is the opposite of empowerment.

If I ever wanted to enjoy my life, I had to stop the show, take off my costume, and walk offstage, even if others wanted to continue acting out the same old scenarios. This is not to say that you won't be blindsided. Life happens. Drama happens. It's how you deal with it that can transmute the latent energy of potential dysfunction into positive actions that support your ultimate goals. Whenever drama rears its ugly head—and it will—do your best to *back away*.

This is a skill you acquire only by practicing it. I speak from experience when I tell you this: even the craziest situation will resolve itself much better if you don't allow anxiety and worry to trip you up on your way to a solution.

However awful it seems in the moment, use your tools, like meditation, therapy, good friends, a hot bubble bath to refocus on all the possibility that does surround you. Disengage, breathe until you can see more clearly, and trust the universal plan. Most of all: be sure to look up from your drama . . . and enjoy the sunset.

YOGA

Drama happens between people (interpersonal), but often, this happens because we create it between us and ourselves, as a reaction to what we think has happened, is going to happen, or may never happen. This is known as presence dysfunction, and it only causes anxiety— even on your yoga mat.

When you participate in your own *inner* personal drama in a pose, it means that either you're berating yourself for somewhere you think you should be but aren't or you're asking your body to express outwardly until you're unstable, moving away from your core and increasing the potential for injury. This can lead to handstand kicks that look more like a bucking bronco.

Today, you want to be a river that stays on track to get to its source and carve out something deeper as it goes. Get ready to flow, Mississippi River–style away from drama and toward your best Yoga Body ever!

Begin with 3 to 5 rounds of your Core Warm-Up.

Chair Pose to Crow

This move will strengthen your core, arms, and inner thighs.

- From your last Downward-Facing Dog, step or hop halfway forward on your mat.

- Roll up into Chair Pose, and reach your chest and arms lightly upward.

    Take 5 breaths in Chair Pose.

- Now plant your hands at the front of your mat shoulder-distance apart, palms flat and fingertips wide and gripping strongly into the mat, middle fingers point forward.

- Lift your heels upward as you bend your elbows straight back. Keep your forearms parallel, not winging out to the sides.

- Creep your knees as high up on your outer arms as you can. You might even make it to the outside of your armpits.

- Press knees in and shoulders out against the legs. Keep your hips low.

- This is a vertical pose more than a forward one; press down into your hands, and round your back straight up away from the hands.

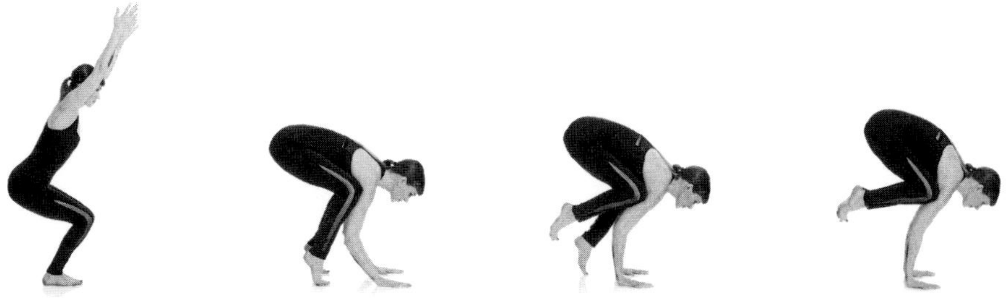

- To fly Crow, look forward (no dropping your head down), and lean your elbows a couple of inches forward—directly over your wrists.
- Lift one or both heels toward your seat. Cross ankles for more power.

  Practice or fly your Crow for 5 breaths! Repeat Chair Pose to Crow 3 times.

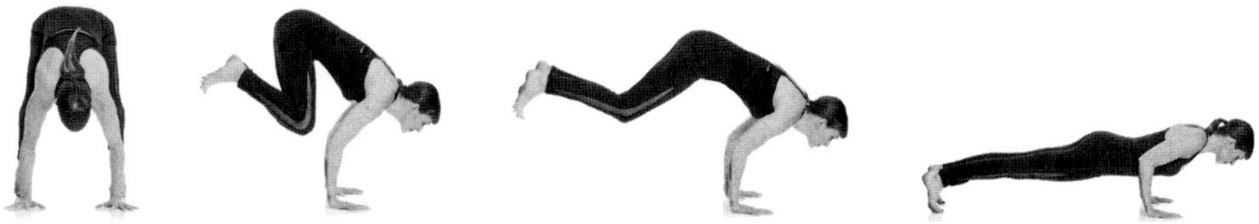

After your final Crow, keep your elbows over your wrists, and either hop both feet back toward Chaturanga or step back into Downward-Facing Dog. Come into Child's Pose for one minute.

When you finish, end with your Core Cooldown.

Namaste! Good job today.

FOOD

Now that you've learned how to start your day off right and mindfully kick drama queen cravings to the curb, you can turn your focus toward choosing meals that are designed to balance your blood sugar.

If the bulk of your diet is simple carbs, not only will you pay with a roller-coaster ride of blood-sugar highs and lows, and the resulting disruption of your energy, but it can cause you to store excess sugars as fat. And did you know that a blood-sugar rush releases the same chemicals as a heroin fix? So you can literally become a carb and sugar addict.

RECIPES

Today's recipes are some of my favorite diet drama-busters. These complex carbs from whole foods satisfy your sweet tooth but roll slowly through your digestive system with the addition of protein, fat, and fiber.

BREAKFAST: ALMOND YOGURT SMOOTHIE

This balanced powerhouse will give you sustained energy all morning. Substitute almond milk, almond yogurt, and unsalted almonds for any other protein in your smoothie. Add a tablespoon of ground flaxseeds and honey for some truly sweet satisfaction.

BEVERAGE: SELTZER SANGRIA

Here's a sweet treat that's also got whole fruit fiber to help moderate the release of fructose, the type of sugar found in fruit.

2 oranges	1/2 cup frozen fruit
1 lime	1 cup seltzer water
half a lemon	

Into a tall glass over ice, squeeze the juice from the oranges, lime, and lemon. Add frozen fruit. Pour in seltzer or sparkling water to fill the glass. Garnish with a lemon or lime slice, and a cocktail umbrella if you have one. Eat the fruit after you drink the water. Substitute white wine for half the seltzer for a fresh, light cocktail.

SNACK: HOMEMADE HUMMUS

One of my staples, hummus contains pureed chickpeas, olive oil, and other goodness, is a creamy mix of whole-food protein, fats, and carbs. I put a dollop of it on many of my salads and use it as sandwich spread, too. You can even add red pepper flakes, pesto, sautéed red peppers, or any other flavor you wish.

2 cups canned chickpeas beans, rinsed and drained	½ clove garlic (optional)
	1 teaspoon freshly squeezed lemon juice
2 tablespoons olive oil or to taste	sprinkle of paprika and cayenne

Put all the ingredients into a blender or food processor. Blend to desired consistency. I like mine a little roughed up, not completely smooth. Transfer to a serving bowl, and garnish with squeeze of lemon and a sprinkle of paprika. Serve with lentil chips or cut veggies.

LUNCH: MANGO SPINACH SALAD

Today, sweeten your salad: use spinach leaves and add half a mango, cut into chunks. Papaya is fabulous, too. Sprinkle with sesame seeds, and toss with your favorite dressing.

DINNER: TRI-BEAN VEGETABLE SALAD

Serves 4 or more

I got this versatile salad from my holistic nutritionist Jenn Pike, RHN, who specializes in keeping her clients sane through delicious food. Make more than you need, and keep some for the next few days. It gets better as it marinates. You'll get so much nutrition and a steady-release blend of carbs, fat, and protein just from this salad that you may not need anything else. But if you want something more, then grill some tofu chunks in olive oil and garlic, or add some organic rotisserie chicken into the mix or on the side.

1 (8-ounce) can organic black beans, rinsed and drained

1 (8-ounce) can organic chickpeas, rinsed and drained

1 (8-ounce) can organic green beans, rinsed and drained

1 (8-ounce) can organic whole kernel corn, drained

4 green onions, chopped

1 jalapeño pepper, seeded and minced

½ orange or red bell pepper, seeded and chopped

½ avocado, peeled, pitted, and diced

1 (2-ounce) jar pimientos

2 tomatoes, seeded and chopped

½ cup chopped fresh cilantro

juice of half a lime

¼ teaspoon garlic salt

¼ cup Jenn's Favorite Dressing (recipe follows)

In a large bowl, combine all ingredients, and toss with dressing until fully coated. Chill in a covered dish in the fridge until ready to serve.

JENN'S FAVORITE DRESSING

I love the suggestion about Mason jars below—I've been putting nearly everything I own in these things. I use pretty Bonne Maman jelly jars a lot.

½ cup olive oil

¼ cup fresh lemon juice

1 clove garlic, minced

1 teaspoon Dijon mustard

1 tablespoon honey or agave nectar

sea salt and ground pepper to taste

Place all ingredients in a glass Mason jar. Shake well until combined.

Store in the fridge. Keeps for up to a week.

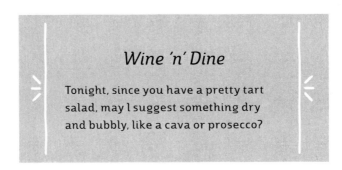

Wine 'n' Dine

Tonight, since you have a pretty tart salad, may I suggest something dry and bubbly, like a cava or prosecco?

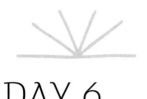

DAY 6

THEME: Act In

I'm going to come out of the emotional closet and hang it all out there for you to see. But, hey—if you can't take the heat, don't write a book.

I used to be totally reactive. Like, high school science project volcano gone bad. I would express my displeasure with other human beings by hurling inanimate objects at them. I remember being nervous around glassware.

Here are just a few of the things I've thrown at people:

∵• enough coffee cups to stock a Starbucks

∵• a freshly baked chocolate cake, stand and all

∵• multiple cell phones, requiring me to buy others

∵• high-heeled shoes (disappointingly clichéd, I know)

∵• an expensive bottle of organic, cold-pressed virgin olive oil (try cleaning that off a tile floor with paper towels)

∵• rings and things

∵• too many swear words to count

When the targets of my explosive anger let me know that my actions were not remotely OK with them, sometimes by leaving the relationship forever, I'd comfort myself with the knowledge that it wasn't my fault: like Lady Gaga says, "I was born this way." After all, I'm Italian and a redhead and a Scorpio six times over. I'd say, "Deal with it. I'm just... fiery."

I'd watch people laugh at Cher slapping Nicholas Cage in *Moonstruck* and then wonder why they couldn't accept it in real life from me. I turned to therapy and yoga—years of each—to try to cool my flame.

Eventually, after lots of practice, I got much better at containing myself through enduring discomfort on the mat and using that energy for something I really wanted (a toned body, inner peace) rather than something I didn't (grabbing the Ganesh statue off the altar and chucking it straight at the too-chatty teacher's head).

More than anything, I wanted to not be "that girl" anymore—the aggressive one who destroys other people's respect for her along with their trust. One day in Savasana, I had an epiphany: I wasn't aggressive by nature. I was, however, completely and utterly full... of bull. I was not genetically predisposed to acting out through violence. I was someone who had gotten used to acting like a child in front of people, and I needed to grow up before I ruined any more relationships, including the one with myself. After all, I was the person whom I mentally beat up the most.

When it comes to reacting to people and situations, some of us act out and some of us act in, just swallowing the fear, anger, and confusion that arise when anything or anyone confronts us. Either way this is not the best we can do.

KARMA

Reaction is the first bunch of feelings that arise whenever something happens that scares or upsets you. Reacting is as natural as jumping when someone surprises you. And you know, no matter how much you practice yoga, compassion, or anything else, you will still experience some reactivity in the face of fear.

The thing that makes most people veer off their center when something isn't going their way is believing that acting from the reaction is the only way to get those intense feelings to go away. It's not that we won't react—we will. It's what we do with those feelings that matters.

Example: if your goal is to manually propel a chocolate cake down the stairs because your mom knew you were on a diet and she made one anyway, then, technically, your actions have matched your vision.

However, if your highest goal really is to be a person of integrity and love, and to represent yourself in the best way you know how out in the world, then perhaps thanking Mom for her baking efforts but politely declining to eat any cake would be a better course of action.

The number one best thing to do when you're about to go all global and postal on yourself or others (unless you're actually mailing a letter overseas) is *absolutely nothing*.

Just for today, instead of reacting, find ways to contain yourself until you can do something that makes you proud instead of powerless. That means no snapping at your kid or your partner, no sending that bitchy first-draft e-mail to your backstabbing coworker, no grabbing for Mr. Jack Daniel's or Miss Marga Rita to calm your nerves.

You'll learn many techniques today to help you learn what to do next, but sometimes the first step in learning how to act is simply not to act at all. So, let's all take a deep breath, count to ten, and get on with what matters most.

YOGA

When I want to gain more lightness and power in every yoga pose, I employ Newton's Laws of Motion.

These laws state that a body in motion (or still) will remain that way unless acted upon by an outside force. The direction it moves depends on which way it's accelerated. And of course, for every action, there is an equal and opposite reaction.

In life and yoga, if you choose to move from fear within, more fear is created outside. If you choose to move from your Core Strength, then that's what you'll get back in your relationships, your daily experiences—and your yoga practice.

To enjoy the benefits of empowering action in a yoga pose, you'll generate extra power with your foundation then contain the ball of energy you created by holding your pelvic center steady, and it will take you where you want to go—lighter and freer.

For example, if you try to hop your feet forward from Downward-Facing Dog with straight arms, it will technically get you there. But you've got no momentum from the actual foundation—your arms—so your legs will accelerate pressure down into the spine, shoulders, and arms, making your pose way heavier. You can't access your Core Strength Muscle Meridian properly unless you bend your limbs first—legs or arms, whatever's on the floor. Then you press down, exhale a squeeze upward into the pelvic and core muscles, and let physics and aligned action lift you upward, decompressing your joints and giving you an experience of your practice that feels inspired instead of impossible.

Today you'll use the floor and Newton's laws by bending limbs, getting closer to the floor, and then pressing down to create momentum that skyrockets a superhero lift through your whole Core Body. This is what right action feels like: lining up with your true potential.

Begin with 3 to 5 rounds of your Core Warm-Up.

Shakti Pulse to Shakti Kick

Now we're really going to have some fun. As you learn to access the hidden power of Newton's laws, you'll tone your arms, Core Body, and courage, too. Start low and slow—and build these over time.

START WITH SHAKTI PULSES

- Press up into Downward-Facing Dog.

- Walk your feet together until your big toe mounds touch.

- Bend your knees, but lift your heels and magnetize your feet together in a bandha, or lock. These actions will engage your deep core arches and inner thighs more.

- Begin to bend your elbows straight back (not out to the sides), forearms parallel. Inhale.

- Exhale, rock your body forward so that the shoulders come over the wrists, and press your arms straight as they root down through the hands.

- As you straighten your arms, lift strongly through your lower belly, and lift the pelvic floor and diaphragm muscles upward.

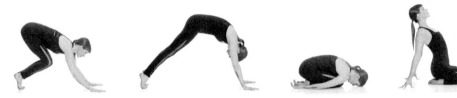

- Do 5 to 10 Shakti Pulses, and then rest in Child's Pose. Sit up, squeeze, and massage out your wrists. Walk your fingertips behind you, and arch your back for a luscious shoulder stretch.

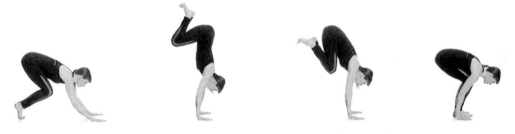

SHAKTI KICKS

It might seem counterintuitive, but you have to bend the arms first to get the most upward momentum as you push downward, yet they end up straight right when you jump. Allow the lightness to lift you through the arms, belly, and legs, in that order, on your strong exhales.

- Come to Downward-Facing Dog. Begin as in Shakti Pulse, but as you press your arms straight, hop your feet off the floor, bend your knees, and draw your heels toward the sitting bones.

- Land lightly on your feet back in a bent-knee Downward-Facing Dog.

- Eventually your hips should hover over your arms, and you'll maintain your hands presssing down and belly lift upward to lightly hop your feet between your hands.

Repeat Shakti Kick 5 to 10 times, and then rest in Child's Pose. Repeat Shakti Kick one more time.

When you're done, on your last Shakti Kick hop feet forward between your hands as if jumping over someone who is lying in the middle of your mat. You can now add Shakti Kicks into any Vinyasa or Downward-Facing Dog if you wish. Then stretch out with Wrist Kiss Forward Bend.

Wrist Kiss Forward Bend

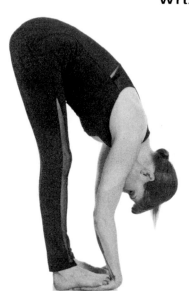

- Separate your feet hip-distance apart.

- Bend your knees, and slide your palms under your feet so that your toes "kiss" your inner wrists.

- Spin your elbows to point toward the shins (not winging out) so that, when you fold, your wrist creases stay straight forward, not twisting.

- Draw your shoulder blades down the back and lengthen your spine.

Take 5 breaths or more in this pose. Release the hands, and roll to stand.

When you finish, end with your Core Cooldown.

Namaste! Good job today.

FOOD

Today I'd like to invite you to keep calm and carry on in the face of life's little and big flameouts. And, as we all know, staying centered is much, much harder if your diet is throwing your system off-balance.

We eat for energy, but our menu can also provide the coolant we need so that stress, inflammation, reactivity, and other fires don't burn out of control, ravaging our inner and outer body with discomfort and disease.

Today's menu supports your intention to pause, slow it down, and cool an overheated constitution by adding many foods that help promote the Big Chill. Eat more of these to calm your digestion, mellow the whole body, and keep yourself on an even keel in this and all other areas of your life.

RECIPES

BREAKFAST: MANGO LASSI SMOOTHIE

In India, they call blending fruit and yogurt a *lassi*. So, I guess this is translated as the "mango smoothie smoothie." It's double-smooth because the ingredients are based on time-tested ayurvedic principles of adding foods like fresh fruit and yogurt to balance too much inner heat.

Use frozen mango and your yogurt of choice today instead of milk or other fruit. A few fresh mint leaves are a great complement if you like the taste. Save half a cup of your smoothie and put it in a freezer-safe covered bowl. Freeze for your snack later today.

SNACK: LASSI PARFAIT

Take out the frozen portion of your mango lassi, top it with some frozen berries, chopped nuts, and granola. Wait a few minutes until it gets more ice-creamy than frozen, and enjoy!

LUNCH: COOLING QUINOA SALAD

Serves 1 to 2

Enjoy my refreshing, high-protein take on the gorgeously fresh Greek salads I had in Santorini.

1 cup arugula

1/3 cucumber, chopped, unpeeled or peeled

1 ripe tomato, chopped

1/4 red onion, sliced

1/4 cup crumbled feta cheese

1/2 cup or so of leftover quinoa

1/2 cup chickpeas or other beans, rinsed and drained

1/4 cup pitted Kalamata olives

1/4 cup chopped parsley

2 teaspoons olive oil

squeeze of lemon or lime

sea salt, cracked pepper to taste

In a salad bowl, toss all ingredients. Put into a pretty serving bowl and eat!

DINNER: MAHIMAHI WITH CUCUMBER-DILL YOGURT SAUCE

Serves 2

This Greek-style dressing is luscious over meat (lamb is traditional), fish, or tofu, and in salads or as a dip. You can make the sauce as the fish is cooking, or do it in advance and refrigerate, covered.

FOR THE CUCUMBER-DILL YOGURT SAUCE

6 ounces Greek-style plain yogurt

1/2 cup peeled, diced cucumber

1 tablespoon chopped fresh dill

1 tablespoon fresh lemon juice

1 clove garlic, minced (optional)

Sea salt and black pepper to taste

FOR THE DILL-LEMON MAHIMAHI

1 tablespoon olive oil

salt and black pepper to taste

2 lemon slices

1 sprig fresh dill

2 (6-ounce) fillets mahimahi or other firm white fish

For the sauce

In a blender, blend all ingredients on Low for a sauce with more texture or on High if you want a smoother consistency. Keep in the fridge in a covered container until ready to serve.

Marinate the fish

In a nonreactive container large enough to hold the fish in one layer, whisk together all ingredients except the fish. Brush the fish with the sauce. Flip it a few times to coat. Cover the fish and put in the fridge to marinate for 20 minutes.

Grill your fish

Preheat the grill, and oil the grate. Take the fish out of the marinade, and pat it dry.

Sear the fish skin side down for 2 to 3 minutes; then flip it, and continue cooking until it's done. The rule is 10 minutes of cooking time for each inch of thickness.

To cook on the stove

Preheat an oiled grill pan until hot over medium-high flame. Follow the rest of cooking instructions above as if for the grill.

Drizzle the whole dish with lime juice and cracked pepper/sea salt to taste.

Top the cooked fish with your sauce, and serve. If you have any salad left over from lunch, some quinoa or sauteed veggies would make perfect sides.

BEVERAGE: WATERMELLOW SMOOTHIE

This cooling concoction is packed with essential vitamins and minerals, full of powerful antioxidants, and tastes totally delicious. l often drink this after a workout.

2 cups cubed ripe seedless watermelon

1 cucumber, peeled and halved

juice of half a lime, plus lime slice for garnish

1 cup filtered or fizzy water

1 cup ice

fresh mint leaves, for garnish

Place all ingredients in a blender. Puree and pour into a tall glass. Garnish with fresh mint leaves and a lime slice. Serve immediately and enjoy!

Spike it: Helloooo, vodka! It's me, Sadie.

ACTION: DOUBLE-DOWN BREATH

Do you know the reason many people feel that smoking calms them down, even though the nicotine in cigarettes is a stimulant? It's the breathing technique that smokers are doing, perhaps without realizing it. When my clients who smoke realize that they've confused the cigarette with their own natural ability to relax, it's much easier for them to kick the habit.

Anyone can do this simple cooling breath. It signals the central nervous system to relax in about thirty seconds, or less, although I suggest doing it for a good two minutes anytime you need to bust an old cycle, a strong craving, or an emotional reaction to help you pause and act in before you act out.

Double-Down Breathing Technique

Sit somewhere quiet.

- Inhale through the nose for 3 slow counts.

- Hold the breath in for 3 counts.

- Exhale twice as slow for 6 counts.

- Hold the exhale for 3 counts.

Repeat the Double-Down Breath for 2 minutes or more. You should now feel more clear, and in control.

BONUS: Three Ways to Act Instead of React

⁖ **The 24-Hour Rule:** Don't respond to a verbal or e-mail confrontation right away, at least until you come to a more stable place. Step away from the keyboard for ten minutes. Get centered enough to match your response to your commitment to integrity.

⁖ **The $50-Plus Pause:** Never buy or commit to anything over $50 if you're buying on impulse. Say "I'll take a little time to think about it." Twenty-four hours later, see how you feel.

⁖ **Put "Yes" on Hold:** When you feel all excited about something, don't say "yes" right away. Take pause, knowing that even a good feeling can mean regrets later. (Many a houseguest has been dreaded this way.)

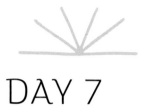

DAY 7

THEME: Three Ts

In 2007, neuroscientist David Eagleman began a series of experiments on the human brain and its perception of time. It wasn't done only in a lab but also at an amusement park. Eagleman's subjects were strapped onto a ride with their back to the ground, looking up into the sky, and then hoisted about 110 feet into the air, or the equivalent of a ten-story building.

Once there, they hovered for a moment, before suddenly plummeting toward the ground; they were caught by a hydraulic slowdown right before they would have hit the pavement. Good times.

Eagleman asked the subjects to estimate the amount of time they were in free fall, and they almost always overestimated the time by about 36 percent. This means that time didn't speed up for them as one might think . . . *it actually slowed down.*

A paper out of Stanford University entitled "Awe Expands the Perception of Time" says basically the same thing as Eagleman, but here the perception of time was triggered not by fear but by inspiration. Both these studies point to what spiritual masters have been saying for centuries: the more present you are to what's happening, the more your life will expand. Simply put, when you pay superfocused attention, to anything, you will think your moment lasts longer than it actually does.

Unfortunately, many people cycle through years of dysfunction, drama, and despair. Their days also seem longer, but it feels more like doing time in prison than being released into the longevity of joy. So the type of reality you're paying attention to matters.

Presence is important, but the *quality* of that presence, like the road less traveled, is what makes all the difference. You are here right now, whenever and wherever you find yourself. But how?

Are you sitting in a yoga class zoning out and not doing your best? Did you walk through a beautiful garden and hardly notice because you and your partner just had a fight? Does money stress keep you from enjoying your kid's birthday party? And all of the moments in between, when it seems like very little is happening, do you just sleep-walk through them?

All of these are examples of what I call "time traveling." You are technically in one place, but your mind has gone warp-speed to some other, to a time which may have already happened, might happen, or might never happen, but it's all probably *not* happening right here and now.

When you time travel, you instantly devalue your present moment from the Tiffany standard it could be down to a bargain-basement level. You, my friend, don't need to be the Dollar Store. If you start to savor each day of your life or, as the writer Rudyard Kipling said, to "delight in the little things," you will soon start really, deeply *living* in the most awestruck ways.

If you want to fall in love with your world and master the art (and, now we know, the science) of being more wholly present in your life, then being aware of the quality of your Three Ts is a surefire way to make it happen more often:

- your thoughts

- your tongue

- your time

Today, we begin to strengthen the skill of mindfulness. You will practice directing your thoughts toward the positive, constructive, and helpful. You'll ensure that your tongue speaks in a respectful, clear, and effective way. You will redistribute your time in a way that serves your highest directives. When you practice high-quality mindfulness the majority of the time, your world will slow down and begin to serve your truth. When it comes to elevating your mind, heart, and days, there's no waiting; there is only now.

YOGA

Some people, especially those who like to push themselves, think a more introspective, cooling practice won't help them move forward with their body, mind, and life goals. In fact, backing off and backing inside are important ways to evolve to your next higher level of being.

These yin poses balance your more yang—or fiery and active— aspects. Going yin reduces stress hormones and dissolves mind and muscle tension, factors that can cause weight gain, anxiety, low energy, and a diminished capacity to rock.

Today as you move through these longer-held positions, slow your breath, and deeply notice the moment at hand. Life's nectar is found inside each sensation, every movement. With endurance holds that build attention instead of muscle, we not only release the body, we train the mind. The longer you can link your deep observation with this moment, the more you'll stretch out your life along with your limbs.

Begin with 3 to 5 rounds of your Core Warm-Up.

Use as little effort as you can to be in each pose in alignment. Allow yourself to receive more instead of working harder. Your breath can even be softer today.

When you finish, move straight into your Core Cooldown. I want you to do the whole sequence as usual, but I am going to add one additional pose and also ask you to hold each pose a little longer than usual:

⁃ Pigeon Pose: Hold 3 minutes on each side.

NOTE: If you want to take it down a notch to practice longer holding, put your knees down in any pose and try to use only your Core Body to do the poses—as if a smaller, more interior, stronger you is moving, not the obvious external physical form you can see. This cultivates a sweet spaciousness between your Deep Core Body and the outer muscles and skin.

- Janu Sirsasana Forward Bend: Hold 2 minutes on each side.

- *NEW:* After your Janu Forward Bend, widen both legs for Seated Fan.

Seated Fan

- Flex your feet with toes pointed toward the sky, and fold forward onto a bolster, stack of pillows, or block under your forehead.

- Now totally relax all your muscles so that you're in a true yin pose—just beginning to feel a light stretch (connective tissue is not meant to strongly stretch, so keep it mellow) anywhere around the joints: knees, hips, and spine.

- Let your back round and your head relax, and breathe into the pose with mindful attention.

Hold Seated Fan for 5 minutes.

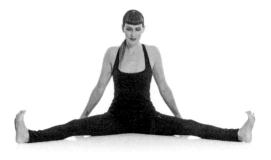 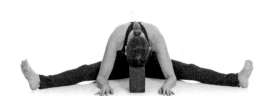

Continue your Core Cooldown.

End with a long, leisurely Savasana, final resting pose.

Namaste! Good job today!

FOOD

Woo-hoo!! Welcome to your healthy hedonism treat day. I want you to splurge and enjoy a little more food than usual and go for the highest Y-Factor you can get (Y for yum, of course!).

Even so, apply the Three Ts to what you eat and you'll become more aware of the places where you can have fun and still nourish yourself with high-quality food. This way, you'll meet your ultimate goals of being core strong, fit, and fabulous instead of always falling prey to the lures of what you want—without respecting what you need. Instant gratification is the death of many a good intention.

As you're approaching the end of your first week of the program, don't forget you can indulge once in a while. And it doesn't always have to be organic and full of nutrition. Have a Sex on the Beach cocktail. Then, hell, have sex on the beach! Eat a whole bag of chips. Whatever. I fully enjoy retoxing what I detoxed now and again. Just keep it in check. Here's how.

RECIPES

BREAKFAST: PEANUT BUTTER CUP SMOOTHIE

The avocado gives this decadent-tasting treat a nice silky texture—and you won't taste it at all, promise. Instead of chocolate syrup, you could also substitute 1 to 2 tablespoons raw cacao nibs for the syrup and organic chocolate coconut or almond milk for your regular milk.

1 frozen banana, halved	1 tablespoon nut butter
1 tablespoon organic chocolate syrup	half an avocado
3/4 cup plain or chocolate Greek yogurt	1/2 cup unsweetened almond or coconut milk
1 teaspoon espresso powder (optional)	additional chocolate syrup and/or cacao nibs, for garnish

Blend all ingredients until pureed, adding a little water if you prefer a thinner consistency. Serve garnished with a swirl of chocolate syrup or a sprinkle of cacao nibs.

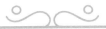

Snacks

Full disclosure: I know snacks. I used to have a huge processed-snack addiction. You name it—if it was found on a gas station shelf, I'd eat it. It's OK to have these things once in a while, but at that time, moderation and I had never even met. Now, when it comes to in-between meals, I full well know you're not going to want hummus and veggies every time. That's fine. Luckily, it's not just a choice between rabbit food and crap.

There is a happy medium out there—snacks that do a pretty darned good job of covering your fourth T: tasty. While perhaps not being the most balanced thing you could eat, these at least are made with whole ingredients your body can reasonably process, not store.

Instead of MSG-laden chips
Try: Deep River "Nacho Kick" chips, Kettle Chips' "New York Cheddar," or Pirate Brand's Smart Puffs with real Wisconsin Cheddar.

Instead of packaged cookies
Try: Paul Newman's Organics—a treasure trove of pure ingredients healthfully masquerading as prepackaged junk food like chocolate crème, ginger, and oatmeal cookies; peanut butter cups; and more. Plus, all post-tax profits go to charity, so you eat well and do good, too. Rest in peace, Paul.

Instead of crunchy snacky things
Try Evol Flatbreads—thin crust, delicious all-natural flavors (that you can store in the freezer) like Italian sausage and caramelized onion or goat cheese and . . . sorry . . . what? I was too busy eating. Or, Smartfood's Buffalo Cheddar popcorn. It's like eating hot wings by the handful!

I could go on and on. Have whatever you want today. Just challenge yourself to snack smarter.

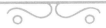

LUNCH: PEARLY GATE TACOS

Serves 1 to 2

I had a version of these at Rosetta's in Asheville, North Carolina, and I thought I had died and gone to BBQ heaven before I realized with a shock that they were completely organic and vegan.

1 cup rice, preferably brown

1½ cups water

pinch of sea salt

½ cup black beans, rinsed and drained

½ cup crumbled tempeh

1 tablespoon organic BBQ sauce

2 crispy corn or soft corn tortilla shells

a few arugula leaves

¼ jalapeño, de-seeded and sliced

¼ red onion, sliced thin

1 tablespoon guacamole and/or salsa

¼ cup shredded cheese

dollop sour cream

Cook your rice in water with salt in a rice cooker or saucepan while you prepare the rest. Stir the beans and tempeh into the rice for the last 5 minutes of cooking.

Transfer the rice mix into a bowl, and mash it together with some BBQ sauce.

Spread a thin layer of BBQ sauce into heated taco shells. Add the arugula, the beans, tempeh, and rice mix next, and garnish with japaleño, onion, guacamole, salsa, cheese, and sour cream as you wish. Serve.

DINNER: CHILI NIGHT!!!

Serves 2 (Unless you ate four tacos. Then, you're good till morning.)

This is my superspeedy way to get some blue ribbon–worthy chili into my face when I'm tired and I don't want to cook.

1 (14-ounce, or so) can of organic chili

olive oil

1 to 2 strips regular, turkey, or veggie bacon

2 cloves garlic, diced

1 to 2 links chicken or veggie sausage, sliced

½ cup shredded organic cheese

¼ red onion, sliced

1 tablespoon plain Greek yogurt

Heat the chili in a pan over medium heat, stirring occasionally until just boiling. At the same time, grill the bacon in a very light coating of olive oil over medium-high heat till browned.

Set the bacon aside to cool on a paper towel, and wipe the pan clean. Reheat the pan, with olive oil added, and sauté your diced garlic. Place sausage slices in with the garlic until browned. Mix the sausage into the chili. Place the chili in a serving bowl, top with cheese, red onion, and plain Greek yogurt, and crumble bacon on top.

DESSERT: STRAWBERRY SUNDAE FUN-DAE

I usually have my double-calorie day on Sunday Funday. Since I used to love a certain fast-food chain's strawberry sundae, though it could probably double as bathroom tile caulk in a pinch, I decided to remake it into an organic dream so that I could use it—not lose it—in my Yoga Body lifestyle.

1/2 cup fresh or frozen strawberries, sliced	3/4 cup coconut milk–based vanilla ice cream
2 teaspoons honey or agave nectar	1 tablespoon chopped nuts of choice

In a small pan over medium heat, warm the strawberries. As they cook, stir in your sweetener, and mash the fruit with a wooden spatula or other mashing utensil.

Transfer the mixture into a freezer-safe container and cool in your freezer for 10 minutes. I like it still slightly warm.

Put your ice cream in a serving bowl, and top with strawberry mix and chopped nuts.

Wine 'n' Dine

The one area where I won't tell you to go all hog wild is alcohol, for obvious reasons; however, if you're going to have one, or even two, today—make 'em count. My favorite wines to drink with chili are big, spicy, chewy reds like Tuscan Rosso or Brunello. This is a great opportunity to have a special glass of wine. And by "special" I don't necessarily mean more expensive. Slow down and savor every sip.

ACTION: THE THREE Ts

Since all you have is now, and all the power you have to transform suffering into possibility happens here, let's employ the Three Ts to help you move into the here and now in a next-level way. Remember, it's not just that you're present . . . but how and why.

1. Thoughts

The biggest roadblocks to rocking your moment are fear-based thinking and its offshoots, like taking things personally and being defensive.

If you watch your body, you are watching your mind. The second you begin to time travel, your body will become anxious. When you feel this disturbance, ask yourself the following questions:

- Is this thought lighting my fire or putting it out?

- Is it providing me with tools I can use to create a solution?

- Is it actually happening right now?

If the answer to any of these is no, see if you can bring your thoughts into alignment with a more expansive or effective perspective. Discern which thoughts create solutions to your challenges and which ones are just getting in the way. Pay all your attention to the former.

2. Tongue

So often, we leak energy through negative self-talk, gossip, not telling the truth, and/or neutral, meaningless chatter. Before you speak, pause, reflect deeply, and then ask yourself:

- Is this deeply, calmly true for me?

- Is it respectful?

- Is it necessary?

- Is it clear?

Do you really need to talk about how stupid-drunk Carol got at the office party? How does it feel in your body when you say things you wouldn't want others to say about you? When your integrity wavers, so does your life force.

How about those times your tongue moves but you couldn't care less about what it's saying. Your words create vibrations inside of you, vibrations that are healing or degrading—and they also ripple out to resonate throughout the cosmos. Wouldn't it be beautiful to paint yourself, and the universe, as a conscious masterpiece?

3. Time

Before you start something, ask yourself:

∴ Do I want to do this?

∴ Is this energizing for me?

∴ Does it move me in the direction of my ultimate goals?

∴ Will this use of my time serve others positively or will it negatively enable them?

∴ Will I feel empowered or disempowered after doing this?

Here's an example of how to use the Three Ts in an everyday situation:

Next time you've **agreed** to be at dinner with someone you love, put down the smartphone, **let your mental marathon rest**, and instead of zoning out, **zone in**.

Listen to what they say, those **precious words of offering** meant only for you, without judgment or expectation. In this moment, there is nothing but love, and love doesn't need to criticize, only to **receive and appreciate**. If **expression** is called for, then do that out of love, too, never out of fear or anger.

So, **look** deeply into this person's eyes. **Notice** the little things: a stray hair resting on the collar because they brushed their hair to look nice for the date or the way they touch their napkin when they get nervous. Really **take them in**, and with them, every-thing that surrounds you. **Tell them** how much they mean to you and how you **adore** that they did their hair to look nice for you, **regale them** with a funny story about your day, **state your opinion with respect** for theirs, and try to **pronounce *bruschetta*** with a real Italian accent.

Seek the magic right in front of you: your glass of champagne, for example, with all its bubbles climbing upward like little monkey babies on a vine. **Feed your date** chocolate mousse.

When you can approach any person, including yourself, or any situation this mindfully, you will finally be invited to open the gift of the present: the ability to approach right here, right now with reverence and then sit back and wonder at the joy that springs up from the cracks in between control.

With practice, refining all Three Ts and the actions that come from them will become second nature.

There's a reason the poet Pablo Neruda wrote a book of odes to seemingly mundane things, like an onion. True artists can fall in love with anything. You're about to develop a huge crush on yourself, everything you see, and the people you choose to keep close to you.

When even a simple saltshaker's top glinting in the candlelight captures your attention, as one is doing before me as I write this, time will slow down. And by a stroke of self-created luck, you'll suddenly have a whole lot longer to enjoy all the facets of your new, delightful life.

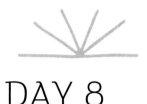

DAY 8

THEME: Rock Who You Are

After one of the first yoga classes I ever taught, a student came up to me and said, "Thanks for class. But I'm used to a faster flow. Do you think you could speed it up next time?"

"Uhhhh...sure!" I said, wanting her to come back again. So next class, I tore through the poses faster than a cheeseburger and fries after a ten-day juice cleanse. Afterward, another student approached me. "Sadie—this class is much too fast for me. Could you take it slower next time?"

The requests continued in much the same vein for the next month: "Talk less!" "I miss what you say! Talk more." "I love your music!" "I can't come back if you don't turn that heathen rock-and-roll music down!" And so on.

I tried to be thirty different teachers in thirty days. Finally, on day thirty-one, I was about to tear my hair out (except I'd just had it done and it was supercute). Instead, I just broke down. Or rather, I broke *through*.

I was so exhausted trying to squeeze myself into so many different molds for everyone else that I wasn't having fun anymore. I wasn't being me. I decided that I'd rather have no one in class than continue to teach like, and for, other people.

So I just walked into class one day and put my iPod on my favorite playlist. Then I sat down, opened my mouth...and shared my truth. Ninety minutes later, I had ten students surrounding me telling me how much they loved the class. I noticed some others who left quietly and never came back, but those ten students returned, and then twenty, thirty, and soon forty to fifty people were joining me in each class.

Each time I taught, I became more courageous and revealed a little more of my voice—my unique perspectives on the yoga teachings—instead of just reading quotes from a book. I soon realized that the satisfaction I felt after fully expressing myself was more important than what anyone thought of it or decided to do with it from there.

As a happy side effect, the more authentic I was in class, the more my "tribe" surrounded me, until my classes were among the most well-attended in all of New York City. I didn't set out to do that—it happened as a by-product of doing my own work.

Perhaps you've been hiding behind the mask of what you think you should be to make others like you or to keep them around. Maybe you're even trying to emulate or please someone else to the point that you're not owning who you really are. This friction between your truth and your actions will cheese grate your soul. Today remember that your point of view, needs and desires, and way of being are just as valid as those of anyone else.

It is freeing to understand this, because now you don't need to take it so personally when someone else disagrees with your truth. Theirs is just another version to choose from. Nor will you believe them when they tell you you're not enough, you're not OK, or they don't think your way is the right way. You can believe them, but you just don't have to. Everyone you meet is holding up a sign to you that says, "Is this you?" It's up to you to seek the answer to that question. Step back, refocus on invigorating your inner flame, and live your own best day. After all, a person won't change, no matter how hard you push . . . unless they can or want to. So stop wasting their time and yours.

Just do you. Spend every waking moment rocking who you are, and everything else you require to be healthy, hot, and whole is coming. In fact, when you rock yourself harder than the Rolling Stones, it's already here. You might not get what you thought you wanted . . . but you'll get what you need, every time, which is far better. (Thanks, Mick.) Now that's a truth we can all get behind.

YOGA

Whenever you are anxious, upset, dark, or sad, you can be sure you've just sold yourself a bill of goods that isn't uplifting and called it "the truth."

We yogis know that truth is relative—you can choose what you want yours to be. "I suck" is one truth, and so is "I rock." They are only two little letters apart, but there's a universe of difference. The most rock-blocking thing you can do is to believe your own limiting stories. So which one will you live out today?

Sometimes when I'm feeling blah on the yoga mat, I switch my truth up and decide to "Be the Yee." This means I must move as if I'm the icon of yoga awesomeness, Mr. Rodney Yee himself. Believing I have the same Yee-like qualities of grace, fluidity, and poetic power instantly improves the state of my body, mind, and spirit. I feel juicy; I feel free. So why not?

On the other hand, your personal reality may be that you have really tight hamstrings. Telling yourself that you're going to "Be the Yee" and push into a too-advanced stretch until something snaps is not a core truth—it's an ego-centered delusion. Know the difference: today in your own poses, create a new truth that empowers *you* and still adapts your postures to respect your current limitations.

Begin with 3 to 5 rounds of your Core Warm-Up.

FLYING WARRIOR FLOW

Warrior II

- From Downward-Facing Dog, step your left foot to the left thumb.

- Ground the back foot down, and roll up through your spine.

- This time, open your back hip and shoulder until you're facing the long left edge of your mat. Your foot might parallel the back edge of your mat, or angle more diagonally forward.

- Lengthen your spine, and unroll your arms out straight forward and back in line with your legs.

- Palms face down.

- Maintain your front knee pointing forward, not knocking in.

- Press strongly through your heels to ignite the hamstrings, draw up through your lower belly and front spine, and look forward with dedication past your front fingertips.

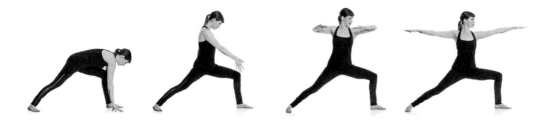

FLYING WARRIOR II TO FIERCE WARRIOR

- Inhale, lift your toes, straighten your legs, and pull energy through your spine and arms as they reach up.

- Exhale fiercely as you bend your elbows, press out through your palms, and bend your front knee into Fierce Warrior and then flatten palms back into Warrior II.

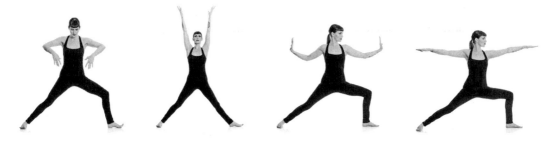

Repeat Flying Warrior II to Fierce Warrior at least 5 times or more.

Triangle Flow

When you come up from the floor in a wave through your Core Body rather than from the linear arms and straight legs first, you'll feel the strength-boosting body-aligning difference right away.

- ❖ From your Warrior II, place your hands back down to frame your front foot.

- ❖ Plant your left hand on the mat outside your left shin or up on a block, or hold on to your shin.

- ❖ Exhale, press feet down, and lift your toes.

- ❖ Keep your front knee bent, lengthen your spine, and start turning your top right hip and shoulder to the sky.

- ❖ Unroll your right arm straight up into the sky, elbow first, as if drawing back a bow and arrow.

- ❖ Now see how straight (or not) you can get your front leg without compromising the alignment of your Triangle Pose.

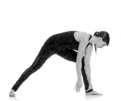 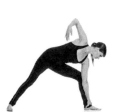 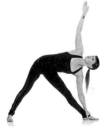

FLOW IT

- ❖ Exhale, and bend both knees—yes, the back one, too. Roll your torso back down, and return your right hand to the floor.

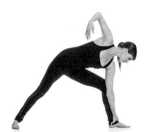 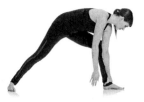

✦ Inhale, and unfurl again into the full pose in a wave from floor to Core to Expression.

Repeat Triangle Flow 3 to 5 times; then hold Triangle Pose for 5 breaths.

Feel free to look down and/or bind the top arm behind your back to de-stress the neck.

When you finish, end with your Core Cooldown.

Namaste! Good job today.

FOOD

BECOME A WINE GEEK

Many people are intimidated by wine, yet when it comes to great wine, and picking the ones that you love, the best expert to trust is yourself. Ironically, a wine expert told me this.

My friend Joe (see below) said that many people who come to him for a tasting instantly stop trusting their own palate, thinking he knows more than they do about wine, which he technically does.

However, authority itself should not make you give over the power

Joe's Wine Tip

Expand your palate and your choices: When you go to a restaurant, take advantage of their custom of letting you try sips of wines before you choose a glass. Don't default to the wine you know you like. Try others you haven't gotten to know, and perhaps you'll broaden your palate along with your library of wine knowledge.

to decide what you like or need. When you walk down the street, do you know whom you find attractive? In a store, do you know what shoes you like? When you see a dinner menu, do you know what you want to eat that night? Sure you do. So now you can tell people which wines you like, or don't, too.

RECIPES

Today I'm offering you room for adventure. I always say, "I don't cook—I create with food." See what you can whip up within this structured freedom.

Before you make breakfast, do some *soji*, the Japanese art of mindful cleaning, and as you clear away and organize anything that needs your attention, make a point of setting your focus on getting rid of any dusty old thoughts, stories, and truths that are cluttering up your Temple of Self.

BREAKFAST: FREAKY FRITTATA

Today, make a frittata, and then tweak it your way. This is a great time to get rid of some leftover veggies from last week!

SNACK: YUMMUS PLATE

Use your hummus creatively today. Garnish it with something delicious, use it in a sandwich or salad, or, hey, brush your teeth with it. Whatever—it's good for you.

LUNCH: MISO HUNGRY

This is my personal take on the classic Japanese soup. Miso soup is legendary for its anti-aging, detoxifying, and digestive optimizing benefits. And it's supereasy to make. Make this meal a mindful miso ceremony.

Your health food store probably has instant miso soup packets, great for the office or in a time crunch; however, fresh miso is superior if you can find it. One tub can last up to a year, so it's a great item to have handy.

1 strip wakame (sea vegetable)
or 1 teaspoon dried wakame
(I often use spinach leaves or
kale in place of the seaweed)

2 cups filtered water

¼ cup assorted veggies, sliced
small (green onion, thin carrot
slices, zucchini, edamame,
peeled and thinly sliced fresh
ginger all work)

¼ cup diced tofu

1 to 2 tablespoons organic white miso to
taste

½ cup cooked brown rice or quinoa
(optional)

If using wakame, soak it in water for 10 minutes and then slice.

Put the 2 cups of water and veggies in a saucepan, and bring to a boil. Reduce heat and simmer for a few minutes, until tender and brothy.

Pour the soup into a serving bowl. Let it cool slightly—a superhot liquid can wreck the enzymes and beneficial bacteria in the miso. When the soup has cooled a bit, stir in the wakame, tofu, and the miso. Add the grain, if desired, and serve.

DINNER: BUDDHA BAR

This name comes from my time spent at Kripalu and Omega, two big mind/body centers here on the East Coast. They always have an area in the café called the Basics or Buddha Bar with a selection of the most unadorned, simply prepared foods. This makes sense. When asked what made him the Buddha, he replied: "Because when I eat, I'm eating." What an aware, mindful dude.

You have a Buddha Bar now, right in your fridge. Tonight, I suggest you keep it simple and practice presence: enjoy your meal as it shares its naked truth with you. Honor that offering of authenticity with pleasure.

Here are some of my favorite ingredients to layer in a bowl, but ask yourself what creation you feel like making. It's probably the one your body wants to eat for a reason. Go, Buddha belly, go!

1 tablespoon olive oil

1 clove garlic, thinly sliced

1/2 cup mixed veggies, thinly sliced

1 cup greens, chopped

1/2 cup cooked lentils or black beans

1/4 cup water

1 cup cooked grain, such as rice or quinoa

handful of nuts

1/4 cup dried fruit

dash of soy sauce, hot sauce, or sesame oil

Sea salt and pepper to taste

In a pan over medium heat, warm the olive oil, and then stir in the garlic and cook until slightly browned. Add the sliced veggie mix and sauté until soft, and then add the greens and sauté until wilted. Set aside in a bowl. Into the same pan, add the beans and water, and cook until the water boils away and the beans are warm. In a bowl, layer your grain, then beans, veggies, nuts, fruit, and seasoning. Stir until well mixed. Serve and enjoy!

DESSERT AND BEVERAGE: BERRY CRUSH TEA

This is a simply lovely way to seal your meal and get more antioxidant-laden tea and berries into your Yoga Body.

1/2 cup fresh or frozen berries

1 cup filtered water

1 tea bag herbal, berry-flavored tea

touch of honey or agave nectar

In a bowl, crush your berries with a fork. If the berries were frozen, let them warm to room temperature. Bring the water to a boil, and brew the tea in a large teacup for 3 minutes. Add the berries to the tea, and any sweetener, if desired. Drink (and eat) up, and enjoy the infusion.

ACTION: THE MAGIC 8 BALL MEDITATION (USE YOUR INSIDE VOICE)

Today, practice some inner sensitivity training. There are three steps to accessing, then living your new, empowering truth out loud so that you can not only know it but be it and attract it, too.

Step 1: Make space and time to listen to your inner voice.

Step 2: Trust that what you hear is worthy and necessary to express.

Step 3: Take actions in words, deeds, and agreements that are in harmony with your truth.

When you skip any one of these, you won't turn your truth into your reality, and it will stay locked inside, like a caged animal, wreaking havoc on you and all those around you. Getting mad-skilled at discerning your inner wisdom is like constantly shaking up an inner Magic 8 Ball until you get an answer from your Core.

Sit in a comfortable seat. One of my favorite meditation places is at a beautiful restaurant surrounded by good food and wine where I can hang with my Moleskine reporter's notebook and transcribe my truth onto paper. Maybe yours is a cushion at an ashram or 5 minutes in your bedroom. Wherever it is, find it, breathe, and begin to listen in.

Ask yourself about some looming decision or challenge in your life. The answers you get will be similar to the ones you get on the Magic 8 Ball:

- Without a doubt.
- Yes—definitely.
- Most likely.
- Signs point to yes.
- Reply hazy, try again.
- Ask again later.
- Better not tell you now.
- Cannot predict now.
- Concentrate and ask again.
- Don't count on it.
- My sources say no.
- Outlook not so good.
- Very doubtful.

If you don't get a clear yes or no, maybe it's not time to know, or maybe you need to dig deeper. You'll know it's your inside voice talking to you when you feel a calm certainty about the answer, even if you don't like it. Truth doesn't need to please anyone—even you.

If your heart feels smaller, your belly tight, or your mind anxious, this answer is more likely coming from your fear, not your truth. Breathe. Relax. Ask again.

Here is my Truth-Finder Exercise—three steps that help you learn to discern your truth from all the other noise you hear inside and out:

Step 1: Take 10 minutes today with yourself and a notebook. On the first page, write "Inside Voice." On the other, write "Outside Voice."

Step 2: Ask your inner Magic 8 Ball a question. Don't push for an answer. Sit, relax, and wait. When a knowing arises in you, write it down on the Inside Voice page. If a sensation of fear or some old story arises, write it down on the Outside Voice page. Just seeing it on paper will help you distinguish between the two more easily.

Step 3: Brainstorm one action you could take to align yourself more closely with that truth. Let's say you asked, "Should I look for another job?" And your knowing said "yes" or even "most likely." Then go online and do a job search today. Take steps to move in the direction of your dreams. See how it feels as you go. (Oh, and as a power-expression mission, you have to go to karaoke night this week. And sing. Yes. *Have* to.)

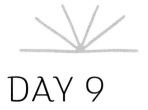

DAY 9

THEME: Clean the Basement

Just as we can only build a home from . . . from . . . sorry. I was a little distracted. Just as we can . . . dangit!!!

I'm sitting at a café, trying to concentrate, and I swear there are crickets in here. Now everyone's looking around, and the more they chirp, the more irritated I'm becoming. I follow the noise back around to my area and tap the guy next to me on the shoulder. He takes out his earbuds, and now he's annoyed.

"Dude!" I snap, knowing with 100 percent certainty that he's the culprit, "do you have a cricket sound on?" He shakes his head. OK, it's not him. Frustrated, I reach down into my bag to get my phone and see what time it is, and guess what? It's. My. Alarm.

Now I vaguely remember resetting my sound to "crickets" a few days ago, thinking it would be a sweet reminder of midwestern nights. In reality, it's more like a car alarm. Red-faced, I turn it off, and now I'm back at work, only with a new realization: that so often, the things seemingly coming at us from others, the frustrations we feel toward the world and the moments that take us off our game, are nearly always coming from inside our own damn bag.

It's only when you have gone inside, and silenced the major dysfunction in the relationship between you and yourself, that you'll stop the inner and outer alarm bells from going off. So why don't more people just open up that bag and turn the cricket off? Our resistance to reaching into the depths of that bag stems from fear.

Big, ugly, scary fear is at the root of all our shadows, just as love is at the root of all our light. When I ask clients what types of dark, heavy, yucky stuff can be found at the bottom of their emotional bags, they cite things like old trauma, fear of loss, lack of confidence, limiting beliefs, and fear of failure. All that stuff could be consolidated into one pile: not enough—the belief that you don't have enough, that you're not enough, that there won't be enough.

If you want to be happy, you've got to open up that bag and let in the light. Yeah, I know. It's probably a terrible time for you to do this today. After all, who looks at their watch and says, "Oh! Three o'clock—what a perfect time for me to revisit my childhood traumas and stress! I'm superbusy, but hey, I can make time to drown in horrible heartbreak again for a few hours." Again, that's fear talking.

You can't protect yourself from feeling by stuffing fear down to the bottom of the bag and pretending it's not there. It *is* there, in most people, scaring you into doing things that limit your Core Strength and diminish your joy. Time to clean it out.

If you can open yourself up to some inner reorganization, you don't even have to know what exactly you're releasing, only that you are ready and willing to do so. The rest will happen organically. When you do get a sweet release, you will feel a clarity and satisfaction that mean you have more fully integrated yourself with who you truly are. Then sit back and watch your outer world do the same.

YOGA

There's really nothing quite like yoga to root out obstacles to your greatness. One of the most powerful ways to cleanse the body is to move mindfully to release deep tension and toxins in the belly and stimulate the digestive system and filter organs, and then invert to sweep any gunk out through the lymphatic system. So I've included some hip-opening, belly-working, and upside-down postures for you today.

Remember, you will gain even more belly benefits by focusing on your heat-generating, root-energizing Belly Bonfire breath.

Begin with 3 to 5 rounds of your Core Warm-Up.

FLOW 1: TEMPLE DANCER FLOW

Releasing deep-hip and pelvic energy requires you to work and open all around the legs, hip joints, belly, and pelvis. These flowing Temple variations will stimulate deeper awakening in your root, removing obstacles and inviting your inner flame to burn brighter.

- Begin facing the left long side of your mat.
- Step very wide, turn your toes out slightly, and bend your knees into Temple Pose.
- Fold between the legs and bring your fingertips to the floor or a block.
- Inhale, and arch your spine.
- Exhale, and curl.

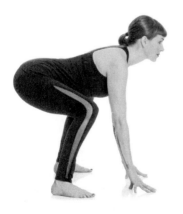 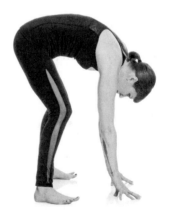

Repeat Temple Arch/Curl for 10 rounds.
After your last Temple Curl
- Press your feet down, and begin to roll up into full Temple Pose.

- Inhale, lift your toes, and pull energy up through your Core Strength Muscle Meridian and unfurl the arms up.

- Exhale, sweep Fists of Fire to your hips, and fiercely say "Ha!"

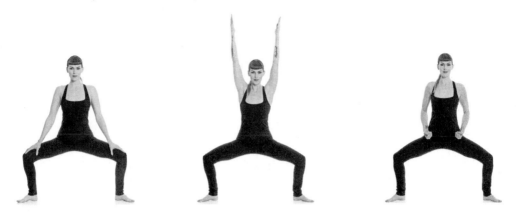

Repeat Fists of Fire Temple 5 to 10 times.

After your last inhale in Temple

- Exhale, and bend your right elbow over your left into Eagle arms.

- Press your forearms together, and wrap the fingers and palms to touch if you can. If not, OK, hey—you're human. Good to know.

- Inhale, arch your back.

- Exhale, curl.

Repeat Temple Eagle Arch/Curl 5 times.

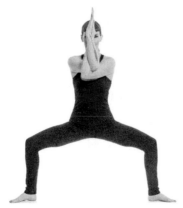

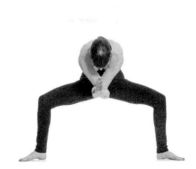

Side Angle Circle and Bind

Here are some uber-hip-opening poses that will release the glutes, hamstrings, psoas, and quadratus lumborum, muscles around the pelvis and lumbar spine that store long-held stress. You'll also clear the shoulder joints with a bind. Got old junk to get rid of? Get ready to have a moving sale.

SIDE ANGLE CIRCLE

- From your last Temple Pose, spin your left toes forward and your back toes in a little. Straighten your back leg so that you're in a Warrior I stance.

- Place your left forearm on your left thigh.

- Circle your right arm back and down.

- Exhale here, turn your chest down, and ground your feet.

- As you inhale, lift your front pelvis in and up, lengthen your spine, and circle your right arm arm forward and up.

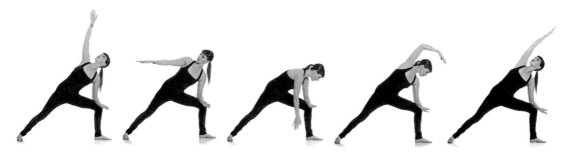

Circle the arm for 5 rounds of breath. Next time your arm lifts, move into Half-Bound Side Angle.

HALF-BOUND SIDE ANGLE

- Bend the top elbow, and thread that arm around your back. The back of your hand will touch your back or maybe even grab onto your front thigh.

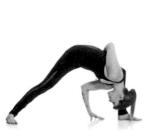 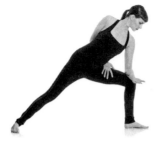 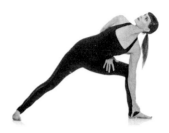

OR TRY FULL-BOUND SIDE ANGLE

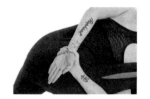

- ❊ Keep your top arm bound, then roll your body down, and curl inside your front leg so that your head faces the floor.

- ❊ Thread your right arm inside and underneath the front thigh, make "OK" circles with your thumbs and first fingers. Try to link them together, or encircle your left wrist with your right hand.

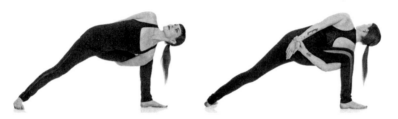

Then move in order through your Deep Core Line to sweep new energy through your basement:

- ❊ Ground your feet down, and lift your toes.

- ❊ Pull your inner thighs up and out the sitting bones.

- ❊ Sweep your front pelvis and lower-back spine in and up.

- ❊ Scoop your sacrum in and up to support your lumbar curve.

- ❊ Wave into a long spine and spin your chest open to the right.

- ❊ Draw your shoulders back, and press your back toward your front knee.

- ❊ Slide your skull back and long so that it rests in one line with your pelvis and spine.

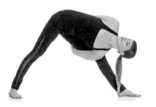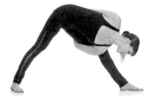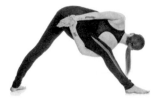

Be in Half- or Full-Bound Side Angle for 5 breaths.

If desired, move your front leg toward straight for Bound Triangle.

Release the bind and end in Downward-Facing Dog; then repeat Temple Dancer Flow and Side Angle variations on the other side.

When you finish, end with your Core Cooldown.

Namaste! Good job today.

FOOD

Today we're going to make your belly even happier. Most wheat and corn in the United States is genetically modified away from its original form, with wheat containing many times more gluten than the original grain, which is why it is thought that people's digestive systems have a hard time processing it.

This is serious business: people are often diagnosed with colitis, muscle and joint pain, chronic fatigue, or Irritable Bowel Syndrome (IBS) when the solution is to remove these foods from their diet entirely or find non-GMO (genetically modified organism), unprocessed sources.

Some people, like me, have celiac disease and cannot tolerate any gluten, which is found in wheat and other related grains, including rye and barley. Some people are allergic, and others simply sensitive to gluten and feel healthier when they don't eat it.

I thought I would flip out when I found out I could no longer have my Italian heritage staples like pasta and bread. Then I got used to it, and I'm happier and healthier than ever (plus I lost twenty pounds of bloat in two months when I stopped). I now take the opportunity to eat closer to the earth and stay away from over-processed foods whenever I can.

Today, we're removing gluten, so here are a few of my simple tips for how to try a gluten-free (GF) diet without giving up your passion for food.

Go Wild: Replace wheat with these grains, ideally in their whole form:

quinoa   teff

buckwheat   sorghum

millet   wild rice

amaranth

Go Whole: Amp up the veggies, fruits, and legumes in your diet. These will give you the energy of carbohydrates but also include a healthy dose of the fiber, vitamins, minerals, and antioxidants your body needs. Aim for organic whenever possible.

Go Home: If it's a challenge for you to find gluten-free or whole food options when you're out and about, make your lunches and snacks at home, or even freeze some in to-go packs, and defrost as needed. There are tons of amazing GF blogs and recipes online.

I'm not big on taking a ton of supplements, because I believe you can get most everything you need from a quality whole-food diet; however, I do take digestive enzymes; probiotics; and omega-3, -6, and -9 fatty acids.

These "big three" can revolutionize the way you look and feel by aiding your belly to properly process, assimilate, and use all the great food you're eating.

RECIPES

BREAKFAST: THE TRIPLE-D SMOOTHIE (DETOX, DIGEST, AND DELICIOUS)

This smoothie packs a huge digestive wallop. The spinach, pineapple, mango, and papaya are full of natural enzymes, and the omega fats help soothe and smooth your GI tract. Digestive enzymes and flaxseed oil are available at health food stores or online. I suggest Udo's Ultimate Digestive Enzyme Blend as well as Udo's Oil.

1 serving digestive enzymes, in
liquid or capsule form (break
open the capsules and shake
the powder right into the
blender; discard the casings)

1 cup frozen papaya, mango, and/or
pineapple

½ tablespoon flaxseed oil

SNACK: THE PRO-PARFAIT

Stir another capsule or serving of liquid probiotics into your yogurt before you build your parfait. You won't taste a thing, but your belly will notice!

LUNCH: BUDDHA BELLY BOWL

Serves 2

Make yourself a power Buddha Bowl that includes raw miso, which is a rich source of enzymes and healthy digestive flora. This is great to make and take with you to work in the morning.

2 cups or so mixed, chopped,
sautéd vegetables of choice

a big handful of wild greens

½ to 1 cup beans or other protein of
choice

1 cup cooked grain of choice

Top with Carrot Miso-Ginger Dressing (page 16) and enjoy the Yoga Body love.

DINNER: BROILED SALMON WITH SHIITAKE-GINGER-GARLIC PILAF

Serves 2

Salmon contains naturally occurring omega oils, and shitake mushrooms, garlic, and ginger may help protect you from digestive cancers. Here's a quick dish that presents beautifully—outside and in.

FOR THE FISH

2 (6-ounce) salmon fillets

2 tablespoons olive oil

juice of 1 lemon

2 cloves garlic, diced or sliced

1/4 teaspoon sea salt

1/4 teaspoon cracked pepper

FOR THE PILAF

1 cup brown rice, Bhutanese red rice, quinoa, or red quinoa

1 cup organic veggie stock and 1/2 cup water (or 1 1/2 cups water if you don't have the stock)

2 teaspoons peeled and grated fresh ginger

1 tablespoon olive oil

1 clove garlic, sliced

1 cup sliced shiitake or other mushrooms

2 cups arugula or raw baby spinach

lemon wedges, for squeezing

sprig of fresh rosemary, optional

Marinate the salmon fillets in the fridge for 15 to 30 minutes in the olive oil, lemon juice, garlic, salt, and pepper, turning once.

Start the rice or quinoa cooking in stock and/or water in a rice cooker or saucepan. Toss in the ginger as it cooks to infuse it with flavor.

Heat olive oil in a pan and sauté the garlic, then the mushrooms. Set aside.

Remove the fillets from the marinade; discard marinade.

Preheat the broiler. Place the fillets, skin side down, on a rack coated with cooking spray in an aluminum-foil-lined broiler pan. Broil the fish 5 1/2 inches from the heat for 10 to 12 minutes or until fillets flake easily with a fork.

When the rice is done, stir in the garlic and mushrooms and any oil from the pan. Season with salt and pepper to taste. Arrange the rice and arugula or spinach on a serving platter; top with the fillets, which will nicely wilt the greens. Serve with the lemon wedges and garnish with a fresh rosemary sprig on top, if desired.

BEVERAGE: THE KOMBUCHA KRAZE

I'm a huge geeky fangirl of kombucha. It is a natural source of digestion-powering probiotics, tastes very tart, is also sweet, and is fizzy. It is available in various flavors like mango, cranberry, and ginger. Some people love it, some hate it, not so many in between. I didn't like it at first, and now I crave it and have one every other day. It's definitely a palate-changer and a game-changer for your digestion. So give it a try.

Kombucha has a very small amount of naturally occurring alcohol, but the effect is more like a gentle mellowing than, say, three hours into a bachelorette party.

ACTION: BOW TO YOUR TEACHERS

Today, can you dig right to the bottom of your bag and lighten your load? What and who are hanging out in there, because you have not yet changed your perspective on the situation and, therefore, cannot let it go? Why are these energies in there? You may tend to blame someone else, and perhaps there's validity to that—not everything that happens to us is our fault.

However, now any emotional baggage you're carrying belongs to you and your responsibility is to find a way to reframe everything from a new loving perspective that will help you finally drop these old, heavy beliefs. If you continue to ignore them, they will stay stuck in you until you realize that they're there to teach you, and allow them to invite you to forgive your past and move on into the magic of your present moment.

Today, sit in meditation with your journal handy. What are the stories that cause you to diminish yourself or live in anger or fear? Can you decide to finally forgive someone who hurt you, that painful teacher, even if that person is you? Not necessarily because you think they deserve to be forgiven, but because *you* deserve to extract all the poisonous barbs from your heart?

Holding a grudge doesn't teach people a lesson or keep you safe. It steals your joy. Let go of the story that you can't protect yourself without being closed and defensive. Open to loving boundaries, bow to your teachers, and walk forward, carrying the lesson but not the weight of holding up that wall.

Bonus Tip: Simple Daily Belly Massage

We all know how the Buddha is depicted: with a big, happy belly meant to symbolize his total expansiveness and inner satisfaction. Or maybe he had a secret stash of doughnuts, who knows? There was a lot of room under those robes.

Anyway, when you're in the shower, in the bathroom, or in bed, relax your belly, and massage it all around with your palms or soft fists. Maybe, like rubbing the Buddha's belly, it will bring you good luck, but it will definitely release tension and stress, toxins and bloating.

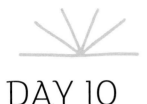

DAY 10

THEME: C'mon, Baby, Light Your Fire

As I write this, I'm at a retreat center on the East Coast to present at a yoga festival. I'm staying in a rustic, comfortable cabin in the woods with bug-screen windows and old-school plumbing. As it happens, I'm in the loo, and let's just say that the plumbing is also taking a restful retreat of its own.

I flush; nothing much happens. I wait for what seems like five long minutes for the water to molasses-trickle back into the tank. When the bowl finally fills, I attempt it again. This goes on six times. Six!!! I'm resting with my forehead on the wall above the toilet, frustrated and annoyed, when I peel my face off the wall, look up, and what's right up here in front of me? A window.

It's about to rain, so the clouds are gathering, and it's rumbling thunder, a noise we hear just about as rarely as "sorry" in New York City. I'm already feeling delighted about that when the shafts of sunlight my mom calls "angel slides" come out through the clouds, beaming down onto the tree just up the hill.

The heart-shaped leaves turn a pale, golden, see-through green, like they just lit on fire from the inside. I forget about how irritated I was just a few seconds ago. Besides, I should be thanking ol' Mr. John here, because if it weren't for him, I wouldn't have been around long enough to catch that perfect moment.

Eventually, John does what he was born to do, and though I'm free to leave the room, I don't want to go. I close the lid and sit down on the throne, like a queen surveying her beautiful kingdom with pride, taking in trees, rain, everything with a new eye, as if seeing it all clearly for the first time.

Yogis call our pinhole views that point us toward suffering *avidya*, or cloudy vision, and it's true. Many people walk around in a fog—veering wildly between happy, coasting by, and distraught—and call it a life.

The opposite experience, *vidya*, clear vision, is like LASIK eye surgery for your soul. The way we get to this clarity, to see the world as a paradise instead of a potty, is to reframe our experience and say "what if" to the possibility that the light you seek is always there, instead of continuing to stumble around in the dark. Part of *svadhyaya*, the inner inquiry, is also filling yourself with light in every way you can, every day.

However, I caution you not to get all fake bliss about it. If someone tells me they never feel angry or irked, I back slowly away from the ticking time bomb. It's possible to recognize that the toilets of life are still there, feel how you feel about that, and then search for the closest available angel-slide entrance. Play there to enliven and expand your heart. Toilet or transcendence: it all depends on where you look. You're not ignoring the negatives. You're simply living the opposite—the only way to transform anything.

Today, seek drop-dead gorgeous, splendiferous love and magic wherever you can. When you become masterful at self-nourishment, resentment and annoyance at life's inevitable malfunctions will lessen and soon hold very little power over you at all.

YOGA

Today we check ourselves into a delight-recovery program. We'll create inner illumination and the metabolic miracle of heat by firing up your deeper core muscles, beyond the often-overused abs.

Specifically, you'll awaken the pelvic diaphragm and sleeping psoas. This way, your spine stays supported, and the outer abdominal muscles will be strong but also supple, available to wholly expand for breath and movement. This is true inspiration: the very act of breathing in, taking in huge deep soulfuls of the sublime.

As you move, focus more on lifting your legs from their actual psoas beginning, higher than the over-gripped hip crease areas. Think of moving your legs from a starting point at the sides of your low-back spine instead. Keep your lumbar spine curve long and natural, and you'll amp up your inner fire.

Also, get back to your Belly Bonfire Breath with a fierceness. I know, it's like Elvis—it has often left the building—but dedicate to the pulsations of relaxing and engaging your pelvic floor and diaphragm as you inhale and exhale. This burns away old ways of seeing the Self and cleans you out to develop a whole new vision. So, get ready to shine.

THE INNER FIRE FLOW

We're going to do one sequence today, repeat it 1 or 2 times, and then enjoy a delicious counterstretching Core Cooldown. Add this flow to the beginning or middle of any of your daily yoga practices for an extra core power boost.

Charlie's Angels Pose

Step both feet as wide as your mat; turn toes out slightly in the same direction as your knees. Bend your knees, and interlace all fingers except for the index fingers. Point them and your arms straight out in front of you for Charlie's Angels Mudra (also known as Jupiter Mudra, the hand position for empowerment).

- Inhale, and bend knees and hips deeper. You can come all the way into a low squat position if you want. If your knees are cranky, stay higher.

- Exhale, and hug and lift your pelvic muscles upward as you root the feet way down and rise higher, about halfway up in the pose. Legs don't straighten.

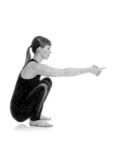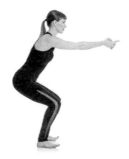

Repeat Charlie's Angels pose 5 to 10 times, with really fierce exhales every time you rise.

End in a Wide-Leg Forward Bend for a few breaths.

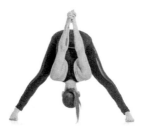

Crossed Boat Pulse

- ❖ Come to a sitting position.

- ❖ Cross your ankles, and lift your knees toward your chest. The balls of the feet rest lightly on the floor.

- ❖ Root your sitting bones, and lift your chest.

- ❖ Make your Charlie's Angels Mudra with your hands, and point it in front of you, between the knees. Or if you are still building strength, hang on behind your knees.

- ❖ Inhale; prepare.

- ❖ Exhale, and lean your body back as you widen your knees and draw them toward your chest more.

- ❖ Inhale as you either bring your feet back to the ground or slide them away from you in the air so that your shins parallel the mat.

✢ Exhale, and hug in again, knees wide.

Repeat Crossed Boat Pulse 5 to 10 times.

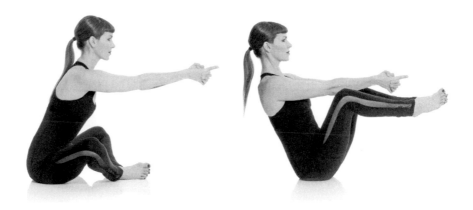

Goddess Boat

✢ Place both feet down in front of you, knees still bent, feet to-gether.

✢ Inhale, widen your knees, roll the pinkie-toe sides of your feet onto the floor. Then, reach your Charlie's Angels Mudra through your legs to stretch the groins and inner thighs.

✢ Exhale, lean back, and bring the wide Goddess legs toward your chest, lifting your feet off the floor.

Repeat Goddess Boat 305 times. Whoops! Typo. That's 3 to 5 times. Now it doesn't seem so bad, eh?

Repeat from Charlie's Angels pose 1 to 2 more times if desired.
End your last round of Goddess Boat by rolling onto your back for Reclining Goddess:

✢ Open your knees to the sides like a book, and bring your feet together.

✢ Place a block under your thighs if they don't reach the ground.

✢ Rest one hand on your chest, one on your belly, and renourish your inner flame.

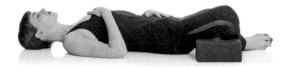

Take slow, gentle breaths here for 1 minute or more.

When you finish, end with your Core Cooldown.

Namaste! Good job today.

FOOD

What most people really want isn't necessarily a faster metabolism but a more efficient one. Have you ever seen a rabbit breathe and twitch? Makes me anxious just being around it. That's a fast metabolism.

"Metabolism" describes the caloric needs you have each day and the systems that break down your food into usable parts, store it as fat or burn it, and help send energy and nutrients to maintain all of your tissues. When your metabolism is working properly, stoked by a clean, full-spectrum diet, you will feel alive and strong, toned and ready to take on the world.

To bring this *svadhyaya*, the inner stoking, into your day on a metabolic level, you also must eat enough: try to starve yourself below your body's basic needs and your supersensitive metabolism will tear down your body for fuel and squirrel away your next meal as more fat. Eat too many calories, even salad and quinoa, and after the body is done fueling muscles and other systems, it will also store those calories.

Today's nourishing meals aim to balance you on your metabolic middle path by giving you enough protein, carbs, and fat to keep you satisfied and focused all day long.

RECIPES

BREAKFAST: THE ALOHA SMOOTHIE

During a recent visit to Maui, I was inspired to create this protein-packed tropical delight for you. It includes macadamia nuts, which are one of the only food sources that contain palmitoleic acid (a type of monounsaturated fatty acid that may speed up fat metabolism).

Today, put a handful of macadamia nuts (organic and raw if possible), some coconut milk or water, coconut flakes, and a tropical fruit, such as pineapple, into the mix. *Mahalo!*

SNACK: FIESTA BEAN DIP

There's so much goodness in this one quick little snack that your metabolism will start to party hearty. This is great taken to work with a little bag of chips or raw veggies. I also make it for dinner (in fact I just did ten minutes ago).

2 teaspoons olive oil

1 to 2 cloves garlic, sliced

1/4 red or yellow onion, thinly sliced and chopped

1/2 cup halved cherry tomatoes

2 cups spinach or other tender cooking greens

half (14-ounce) can of organic refried beans

2 tablespoons organic salsa

1 tablespoon Greek yogurt

1/4 cup shredded cheese

a few drops of hot sauce

Drizzle the olive oil into a hot pan. Wait till one piece of garlic sizzles in the oil, and then (this next part goes fast, so get ready!) sauté the garlic till a little browned. Add the onion and cherry tomatoes, and cook until slightly browned and mushy; slide them to the side of the pan, and cover with a mound of spinach to wilt. Stir once.

In the space you just made, dollop the refried beans. Spread the beans as thin as you can so that they heat up quickly. Stir for one minute or until warm.

In a bowl, layer your beans, veggie mix, salsa, Greek yogurt, and cheese. Garnish with hot sauce if desired, and serve.

LUNCH: HIGH-PRO GLOW

This is adapted from a salad I order all week long while at the sunny Amansala retreat center in Tulum, Mexico. My friend, owner Melissa Perlman, was kind enough to give me the recipe for their most popular dressing.

The pumpkin seeds are high in zinc, which aids in protein metabolism. It's such an easy and versatile dish with a beach-body-maintaining yet sweet dressing that I bet you'll crave it as much as I do!

AMANSALA SALAD WITH HONEY-BALSAMIC-GINGER DRESSING

FOR THE DRESSING

¼ cup olive oil

¼ cup balsamic vinegar

2 tablespoons honey

2 tablespoons soy sauce or wheat-free tamari

2 tablespoons sesame oil

1 quarter-size piece fresh ginger, peeled and cubed

FOR THE SALAD

2 cups spinach leaves

1 cup cubed papaya or mango

¼ cup pepitas (shelled pumpkin seeds)

6 ounces cooked fish fillet or other protein, cut into bite-size pieces

1 teaspoon minced fresh cilantro or parsley leaves

¼ cup sliced scallions

Put all dressing ingredients in a blender, and blend until smooth. Put in a jar or bottle. Keeps in the refrigerator for up to a week.

Toss together all salad ingredients.

Pour out 1 tablespoon of dressing into the salad, and toss. Serve. Gracias, Melissa!

DINNER: EASY CASHEW STIR-FRY

Serves 2

This is something I've made for years; it's a fast and filling standby. I find myself currently wok-less, so I make it in a nonstick pan.

IN RICE COOKER

1 cup grain

pinch sea salt

IN PAN

2 teaspoons wheat-free tamari or
soy sauce

3 ounces organic meat, chicken,
fish, or vegetable protein, cut
into strips

1 tablespoon olive or other cooking
oil

1 clove garlic, sliced

2 cups assorted stir-fry veggies, chopped
to roughly the same size (I dig
asparagus tips, broccoli, red bell
peppers, onions, and mushrooms for
this dish)

1/4 cup cashews

cracked pepper or red pepper flakes to
taste

a few shakes sesame oil

In a nonreactive bowl, toss the tamari or soy sauce with your protein, and let stand for 5 minutes. Drizzle olive oil into a large nonstick pan, and heat to medium-high. Sauté garlic till lightly browned, and then stir in the protein and sauté until browned. Add the veggies, and sauté for 5 minutes.

Remove the pan from the heat. Mix in the cashews, pepper or pepper flakes, and a few drops of sesame oil. Transfer cooked grain to a serving bowl, and toss with a few drops more of sesame oil. Scoop the veggie mix on top of the grain, stick two chopsticks into the dish (pretty!), and serve.

BEVERAGE: GRAPEFRUIT MOCK-MOSA

Grapefruits are notorious metabolic fire-starters. You don't have to go on a grapefruit diet in order to gain the benefits. Just drink up!

8 ounces seltzer water

juice of half a Ruby Red grapefruit

1/2 lemon, thinly sliced

Put some ice in a tall glass. Fill the glass three-quarters full with seltzer, pour in the grapefruit juice, and garnish with lemon slices in the glass and on the rim.

Spike it: Instead of seltzer, substitute prosecco, champagne, or cava.

Since I don't like my drinks very sweet (I'm sweet enough), using my finger I ring the rim of the glass with agave nectar, then dust a salad plate with sugar, and just press the upside-down glass into it. Voilà!

ACTION: FIVE ALIVE

It's too easy to help rock other people's worlds and forget about your own. One of the best ways to blow off those clouds over your spirit eyeballs is to turn toward that which infuses you with joy. Don't wait one more second to do this. Today, list five things that light you up and would put more *life* back into your life.

I asked an artist friend of mine what his "Five Alive" were, and he said, "Doing my work (photography), going to see other artists' shows for inspiration, spending time outdoors, being with the great friends I've cultivated, and having good food and wine." He decided to make a special effort to go to a good friend's party out in a park and take photos to commemorate the event, while eating and drinking great food. Four out of five at once! Well played, sir.

More light-giving possibilities that come to my mind are

- Wear golden cheek shine. You'll sparkle all day long.

- Take lemon-cucumber-infused water with me so that I stay hydrated and bright.

- Plan a movie night with friends. See a funny one. Laughter is lightening.

- Spend one sweet, focused hour on your next creative project.

- Search for "cute kitten" or "best marriage proposal" on YouTube . . . and instantly feel better.

- Flirt (even if you're coupled or married, you're not buried).

- Sweat for at least 20 minutes. (I'm not gonna specify how.)

Make your list of big and little ways to light it up, and then do all of them today. It might seem impossible, but with a broader perspective I bet you can make it happen.

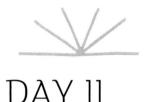

DAY 11

THEME: Yoga Ninja

My ninja teacher is awesome. Sure, his name is Jeff, but he understands why we're going to just go ahead and call him the Ninja from now on (because it's just so awesome).

I don't have a lot of time to go and train with the boys at the dojo, so the Ninja and I struck a deal: we meet, he teaches me a few moves for self-defense, and then we drink a margarita. Two, actually. That's right. Incapacitation and tequila are two tastes that go great together.

How do I feel directly following our meetings? Let's just say that Bruce Lee has nothing on me. The experience of, as the Ninja says, "keeping your peace intact," no matter what someone else decides to do, is quite invigorating.

It's the best time ever, and I highly recommend that you consider finding a martial arts or self-defense class to complement your yoga practice. The only bummer about being a ninja is that Jeff has got all these skills and bits of knowledge, but he never uses them. Dude's been in training since he was fifteen and he's been in exactly zero fights.

The ninja code states that being able to contain all that power is what makes you strong, not using it all willy-nilly. As much as I'd like to grab the next guy's hand that pats my booty at a club, twist it just so, and cause him to kneel down before me in excruciating pain, all while I scream "KARMA, BABY!!!" I realize that this is not the ninja way.

Theirs is a Zen philosophy, one that sees energy not as some elusive substance that everyone wants more of but is too tired to go get, but as a living force that can be conserved, directed, and then used—but only when absolutely necessary. You, too, have the capacity for ninja-like secret inner strength and the kind of live-wire energy usually reserved for people who drink boatloads of caffeine.

People ask me how I got to be as happy, passionate, brave, and successful as I currently find myself. Did Lady Luck smile upon me? Do I have rich parents? Some kind of magnetic power that other people don't have? No, no, and more no.

I designed my life to be something I'm proud of, step by step, day by day. I always say, "Being me is a full-time job," and I mean the type of full-time job that's got a lot of overtime hours but also a lot of payoff. I called upon my power to be consistent in action and direction to keep trekking onward toward my dreams most of the time.

Yogis call this "dedicated practice." You're always practicing something. The question is, what is it? Roadblocking or rocking? Are you practicing actions that take you in the directions you want to go? Every day is another chance for you to hold a thousand dedication ceremonies to your own health and passion. So, what will you tackle today? I'm seated at my favorite Austin, Texas, coffee shop now to throw down and write this book. Then I'll head to a studio and teach fifty people yoga for three hours. After that, I'll head to Texas BBQ at a vineyard with a very cute friend. Book, yoga, wine, 'cue, flirting. My kind of day.

This lifestyle builds your energy instead of depleting it. But get ready: Know what some people will say you are when you finally start taking some of that hard-earned energy for yourself? Selfish. Don't pay the haters one more minute of your attention. They may not yet know the difference between *selfish* and *self-centered*. Selfish is defensive and imbalanced, never giving out, only taking in; self-centered on the other hand is healthy and necessary.

You're self-centering: investing in your own chi, or life force. Approach your energy as the most precious resource in the universe, the original source of you feeling good and living a high-quality existence, and you'll begin to dedicate its use much more wisely. Then you, too, can call yourself a Yoga Ninja. Begin now, Grasshopper.

YOGA

We all have a ninja within. The inner ninja is your self-possessed confidence, the ability to be clear about your truth and stick to it through tough times, and the skill of calm, alert presence. All these states of being arise from an empowered inner relationship, and they are magnetically attractive.

Physically, this aspect of being present with quality and then acting from your core integrity is represented by the psoas muscles, the only ones that bridge your legs (foundation, present moment) to the spine (core, center of Self).

The psoas's path from the inner thigh to lumbar spine (by way of the front pelvis) is truly one of your most profound sources of Core Strength and spinal stability. Today, you'll power up the psoas, let it help stabilize your lower back, and be transformed into the mystical ninja you already are . . . and always were, deep inside.

This is going to be fun. I'll include some sweet moves taught to me by Victor, a great martial artist/yoga teacher in Tulum, as well as by my teacher Jeff Christian. Shout out to my ninja!

FLOW 1: KUNG FU FLOW

This is a unique sequence that will cross-train your regular yoga practice, use your core "pso" powerfully, and allow you to express your true fierceness through sound. Get ready to roar! Hold each pose for 1 to 5 breaths unless noted otherwise. You can start slower and work up to a faster, more Bruce Lee movie look.

- ⁘ Come into Temple Pose facing the left long edge of your mat, toes angled out, knees bent.

- ⁘ Exhale in Temple Pose.

- ⁘ Inhale, turn your right foot forward, and open arms into Warrior II.

- Exhale; slide your back heel back a little, front toes more forward, as you punch your left fist forward and bring the right fist to your hip. Say "Ha!" for more core activation.

- Inhale, and slide your hands past your belly as if carrying a ball of energy from there then reach arms up into the sky. You're now in Warrior 1.

Then continue to Flow 2.

FLOW 2: NINJA FLOW

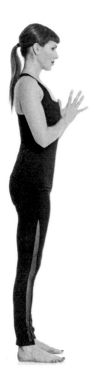

Whenever you use your psoas and transverse abdominis (front top pelvis and front lumbar drawing into the body and upward), you're doing the action I call Ninjasana. You can apply Ninjasana to most yoga poses to support the lower back curve to stay natural.

Use Ninjasana always, but even more in poses that pull your lower back into too much curve—like Chaturanga, handstand hops, or any transition between postures—so that you don't default to overusing your lower-back curve to do your practice.

Begin in Mountain Pose.

- Stand loose-limbed here, feet hip-distance, knees slightly bent.

- Feel your center of gravity at the center of the pelvis.

- Place your hands just in front of your belly, and close your eyes to sense the energy emanating from your core.

Ninja Stance

- Open your eyes, and begin to lean your hips backward so that you almost fall backward.

- Catch yourself by stepping the back foot behind you, parallel to the back of the mat; the knee bends. Your front foot still points forward. Now you're in a Warrior II-ish stance, except the back knee is bent and more weight is on the back foot.

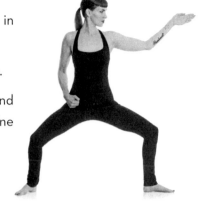

- Make your left hand into a blade: fingers together as in Warrior II, but face the palm to the right, elbow bent.

- Your right hand makes a fist and comes to your back hip.

- Really press open your hips and front knee, shoulders, and arms as if you're a book opening wide from your front spine outward.

Take 5 breaths here, Ninja.

Kick of Fire

Kick anything that doesn't serve you out of your kick-ass life.

- Turn your back heel up. Reach your arms into High Lunge.

- Inhale, and step the back foot forward a little.

- Exhale, sweep your right knee into your chest, and come to stand as you kick out through your heel, leg long and parallel to the floor (hello, psoas!)—and yell "Ha!"

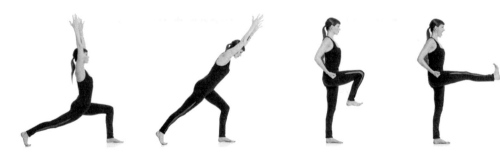

- Inhale, touch the lifted leg back on the mat a couple of feet; arms reach up.

- Exhale, kick again. Keep your front spine and hips drawn back over your standing foot as you kick, not leaning forward.

Repeat Kick of Fire 5 to 10 times. Get loud and proud!

Kung Fu Panda

This pose takes you back to your wild, true nature: a brilliant blend of fit and fierce.

- Exhale from your last Kick of Fire, step back into a deep Temple Pose turned to the side of your mat. Put your paws up, and roar like a Kung Fu panda. Take 3 panda breaths here; growl on each exhale.

- After your last panda roar, turn to stand at the front of your mat in Mountain Pose.

- Exhale superslowly, and as you do, "push" energy down with your palms from your chest to your hips, as if you had your palms on top of two floating beach balls and were pushing them toward the earth. This will seal your energy and close the sequence.

Repeat the entire sequence from Temple Pose on the other side.

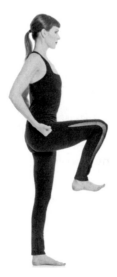
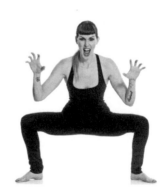

When you're ready, move into your Core Cooldown.

Do all your cooldown poses, but hold the following poses for at least 1 minute on each side today to really release the psoas:

- Pigeon Pose

- Side Janu Sirsasana

- Bridge Pose, or Full Wheel

- Sacral Reset Pose

- Supine Goddess

Namaste, Ninja! Good job today.

FOOD

In honor of discovering your inner ninja superpowers, I want you to fuel yourself with superfoods. Pretty much every whole organic food that exists as nature made it is a superfood—but these are some of the best.

They help protect you against diseases, boost a sluggish metabolism to an efficient level, sweep away toxins, and basically keep all of your systems working to ensure you look and feel your best. This all adds up to unleashing massive amounts of energy for you to use to walk your own path more completely. Prepare to feel superstoked instead of superdepleted!

RECIPES

BREAKFAST: TRIPLE-BERRY SMOOTHIE

Berries are jam-packed with immunity-boosting antioxidants and fiber. Get your berry on this a.m., and boost your energy levels all day long.

Add to your smoothies 1 cup frozen mixed berries and a scoop of protein or meal powder to counteract the fruit sugars. Blend, and serve with a swirl of honey on top.

SNACK: GRAPEFRUIT AND WALNUT PLATE

These are two superfoods that taste great together.

> 1/2 grapefruit, peeled and sectioned
>
> 1/4 cup chopped walnuts
>
> drizzle of honey to taste

Arrange grapefruit sections on a salad plate, and sprinkle with walnuts. Add the honey last.

LUNCH: SKILLET SALAD OR REGULAR SALAD

Use any leftover dressing you have. Boost it with superfoods by adding some or all of the following:

- a darker green, such as spinach, arugula, collard, or kale (if you have time, dress the fibrous kale in a little olive oil, sea salt, and lemon juice and let set for 30 minutes first to soften)

- tangerine or citrus fruit of your choice

- 1/4 cup nuts

- 1 teaspoon ground flaxseeds or chia seeds

- 3 ounces protein of your choice

DINNER: RAW PAD THAI

Serves 2

This crowd-pleaser is courtesy of my nutritionist, Jenn Pike. I love it, as do her kids. The amount of fresh veggies you'll get in this one meal makes it a Core Strength superhero dish that should go into your regular rotation.

The noodles are made from zucchini, but if you love the traditional pad thai rice noodles, you can make some of both and mix them together. This stores well and is perfect for taking to work the next day.

2 medium zucchini, julienned or made into noodles using spiral slicer

1 large carrot, julienned

1/2 cup thinly sliced red onion

1/2 red pepper, seeded and thinly sliced

1/2 yellow pepper, seeded and thinly sliced

1 cup slivered red cabbage

1 green apple, julienned

3/4 cup cauliflower, finely chopped

1 teaspoon fresh cilantro, chopped (optional)

3 tablespoons shredded coconut

ALMOND CHILI SAUCE

3 tablespoons honey

juice of 1 lemon

2 small cloves garlic

4 tablespoons low-sodium soy sauce or wheat-free tamari

1 die-size piece peeled fresh ginger

1 teaspoon salt

1/4 teaspoon cayenne

1/2 cup almond butter

1/2 cup water for thinning

Chop all vegetables, and mix all ingredients together in a large, shallow serving dish.

Place all sauce ingredients in a blender, and blend on Low until smooth.

Pour sauce over vegetables just before serving. Toss and enjoy.

BEVERAGES: POMEGRANATE-LIME FIZZY

Get more superfoods into your diet and superhydrate, too.

2 lime slices, round and thin

3 ounces sparkling water

3 ounces organic pomegranate juice

juice of half a lime

Place the 2 thin slices of lime around the inside of a tall glass to make it pretty. Add ice. Fill halfway with sparkling water and the rest with pomegranate juice. Squeeze in the rest of the lime juice and serve.

THE NINJA MARGARITA

Forget about just being skinny, girl! Let's get superfit and healthy instead. We'll sneak-attack toxins with this low-cal, high–vitamin C margarita. It's chock-full of living foods and nutrients—not preservatives and sugar.

1 ounce clear tequila (I prefer the distilled, no-water organic, Dulce Vida; a little goes a looong way, comprende?)

1/2 ounce Cointreau or Grand Marnier

1/4 cup fresh-squeezed orange juice

juice of half a lime (or 2 tablespoons fresh lime juice)

1/4 cup seltzer or club soda

1/2 cup ice

If you want a salty-sweet surprise rim, take two small plates, and squeeze some honey or agave nectar onto one and a little sea salt onto the other. Turn the glass upside down, stick it in the sweet plate, then the salty. In a blender, combine all the ingredients and pulse. Pour the mix into the glass. Or have it unblended, over ice.

ACTION: CLARIFY YOUR CORE MISSION STATEMENT

It's time to unfold the most important road map of your life. What are your Core Missions? They are the jewels you keep in your pocket, the arrows to help you hit any target. These are not only states of being but *states of doing*—actions you must commit to living out in the world if you wish to feel the uncommon floating lusciousness of having no separation between who you truly are and what you do.

You will revolutionize your life whenever you minimize the gap between your personal truth and your actions. When you do the following exercise, you'll collect a few orientation points to help you scale the mountain of questions about the direction you want your life to take. You'll have a higher vantage point from which you can survey your whole life and see what you've been designing so far and where you want to go from here.

Make a list of up to twenty Core Missions; then see if any of those can be further consolidated into a more concise statement of purpose. Here are some of my Core Missions:

- to treat all beings, me included, with as much kindness and respect as I can and still stay balanced

- to live with both purpose and passion

- to express my personal integrity through action (know what integrity means to you: loyalty, courage, nourishment, humor, self-knowledge, self-love, and so on)

- to say yes to love that's healthy, available, and grounding for me

- to love with my whole heart—especially with regard to myself

- to continue studying and deepening my craft

- to seek adventure and magic wherever I can find it

Let's say some guy came up to me at a party. He's cute as heck and seems interesting, but he just got out of a relationship a few weeks ago and he's "scared to love anyone again." When he asks me out for the following night, I check in with my Core Missions and stop at "to say yes to love that's healthy, available, and grounding."

So I say, "Thanks, but I don't think so." I know I'd rather wait until someone walks into my life already having done their work and steps up with an open heart from the start. Because, honey, I want someone who comes correct. Maybe it will even be him a few months down the line.

Having your Core Missions firmly in mind and heart can save you endless hours of struggle, misalignment, and constantly being in fix-it mode. Drop the people projects, get back to living your Missions, and require that anything you draw close to you be doing the same.

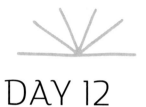

DAY 12

THEME: Date Yourself

And by this, I don't mean that the next time some handsome twenty-year-old bartender makes a *Star Wars* reference you say, "I remember sitting in the theater when I was about your age watching the original movie!"

As anyone who is both prosperous *and* happy knows, it's not enough to have outer success if your inner life s-u-*sucks*. They understand that in order to be truly loved—as well as to love life, other people, or anything else—they must do one central thing: cultivate a lifelong love affair with themselves.

When I say *affair*, I mean it. Most of us are frenemies with ourselves at best. Maybe some of us have attained close friendship, and a very rare few are in total, head-over-heels love with their red-hot self.

Think about it: do you have an inner love-hate relationship? Are there times when you berate, criticize, and diminish yourself? Honestly, if you asked your romantic partner, "How do I look today?" and he or she replied, "Oh my gosh, you look like a huge, fat pig, and you're totally disgusting," you'd probably DTMFA (dump the mofo already). Yet how often do you say similar things to yourself? Do you have a Soul Mate Requirement list in mind, a *manifesto* or *womanifesto* that you want your romantic partner to live up to, qualities like loyalty, a great sense of humor, forgives your faults, and loves you unconditionally?

Then ask yourself: Are you being these same things between you and you? Do you spend quality time with yourself? Do you love being solo *as much as or more than* with any other human being? If you're straining to get some external lover to be your everything and warm you so fully that you need no other light source, I'm sorry to tell you this, but you're heading for heartbreak. You can only give or receive love outside to the extent that you can give or receive it inwardly. There is no other way to attain true love except from the inside out, and if you try, you'll suck the love right out of any situation. So, let's reverse the flow. Today is a true love-*in*.

The best way to begin is to look at the places where you are still having a dysfunctional core relationship and target them for improvement. The feeling of abandonment you might feel in relationships doesn't actually come from the other person. It comes from you, abandoning *yourself* for the sake of another. This is the foundational anxiety that arises when you walk away from loving yourself.

You don't want to stay with a toxic partner, someone who is constantly creating an emotional void that you keep falling into, but regardless of what you decide to do about the other person, start by refusing to abandon yourself, and watch what happens. You will reclaim your power, for starters. No more worrying, obsessing, overpleasing, or contorting yourself to fit into someone else's needs. It's over.

Begin, this instant, to fully inhabit your own heart. Stop putting excess energy toward figuring out how to attract people, how to change them, or what you need to do about any outer relationship.

Today, I want you to pour all that love you have to give back into yourself. You have all the tools at your disposal to become the best friend, mother, father, lover (some of the tools here are literal) that you've ever had. I'll give you a little how-to advice at the end of this chapter, but for now, let this sink into your heart: just for today, give up on grasping on to outer love and get back to doing you.

YOGA

Today we aim to inspire, strengthen, and refresh not just your physical heart but also the yogic aspect of loving compassion, which is the first step toward cultivating dynamic, functional relationships with yourself and others.

In Chinese medicine, your Heart Meridian runs through your hands, arms, and chest. If it's blocked, you will tend more toward anxiety, depression, sadness, even heart disease. Today, we work to unblock and flow energy to your spiritual and physical heart to give it some holistic, rebalancing TLC.

Begin with 3 to 5 rounds of your Core Warm-Up.

Bridge between poses or sequences with a Vinyasa flow whenever you wish.

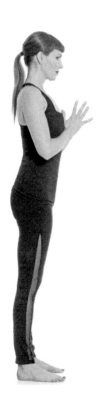

Eagle Pose

This opens the back of your heart, freeing you from past heartbreak.

- ✣ Stand in Mountain Pose.

- ✣ Lift your right knee to cross over your left.

- ✣ Press your shins together and maybe wrap your top foot around your bottom ankle.

- ✣ Bend your arms, and cross your right elbow over your left arm. Wrap the forearms and/or hands around each other.

- ✣ Lift your elbows higher, drop the shoulders, and sit down lower.

- ✣ After a few breaths begin to fold forward into Low Eagle, elbows toward the front of the knees.

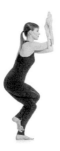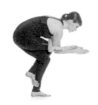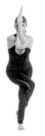

Hold Low Eagle for 5 breaths.

Twist of Fire

- ⭄ Unwind your Eagle and step feet together for Chair Pose.

- ⭄ Exhale, sweep your palms together, and touch your left elbow to your right knee.

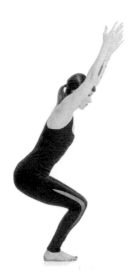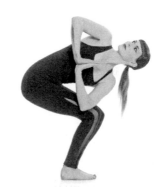

- ⭄ Inhale, float back into Chair.

- ⭄ Exhale, twist your right elbow to the left knee.

Repeat Twist of Fire for 3 to 5 breaths.

Twisted Chair to Side Crow

- In your last Twisted Chair, to the right, begin to lower your hips toward the heels.

- Dig your left arm a little farther around your right thigh.

- Lean forward, and plant your hands on the floor. Hands and arms are placed as in Chaturanga: shoulder-distance, bent elbows.

- Play with leaning into your hands and lifting your heels and hips higher.

- Walk your feet over in a line behind your left hand until your chest is centered between your hands.

- Slide your head, chest, and elbows forward; press your hands down, hug your right knee onto your left elbow, and perhaps fly into Side Crow. In the full pose, you're balancing on one arm, not both, which can misalign your shoulder joints.

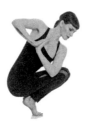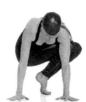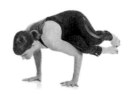

Try or fly Side Crow for 2 to 5 breaths.

After Side Crow, roll back up into Mountain Pose, and repeat Eagle Pose, Twist of Fire, and Side Crow to the left.

After you're finished both sides, interlace your fingers behind you with palms facing, and take a Forward Fold with bound hands for 10 breaths to stretch the chest and shoulders. Breathe into your everlovin' heart.

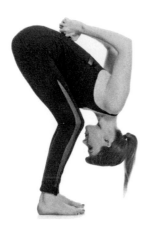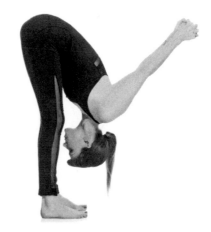

End with your Core Cooldown.

Namaste! Good job today.

FOOD

FAT FREE-DOM

Fat in the mouth does not necessarily translate to fat stored in the body. Although some fats (like transfat) can cause diseases and obesity, eating little or no fat at all can also be a recipe for health disaster. I used to eat a fat-free diet, and I felt life-free, too—like a dry, brittle haystack. And, oh, God . . . my hair, my skin, my poor organ functions. So sorry, brain!

Fats are essential to making your body work, and, paradoxically, you need dietary fat to tell your body it can release and burn stored fat. Many of the world's healthiest cultures eat a diet higher in whole-food fat. It's not avoiding fats like the plague that makes us healthier or less likely to store excess weight. It's eating the right kinds within a balanced diet. Let's add the right amounts of whole-food fat to your diet today and along with it, more whole body love.

RECIPES

BREAKFAST: SILK CHOCOLATE SMOOTHIE

Chocolate plus fats will make your hair, nails, and skin look silky smooth(ie), too! Today use chocolate-flavored milk, or add 1 tablespoon cacao nibs and chocolate protein powder. Add half an avocado, peeled and pitted, to the blender. You're gonna love it.

SNACK: DOUBLE DOWN BEAN DIP

Eat with lentil or corn chips or sliced veggies!

2 tablespoons refried beans

2 tablespoons hummus

half an avocado, pitted and sliced

sprinkle of sea salt

1/4 cup shredded cheese

In a snack bowl, layer the cold beans, hummus, avocado, salt, and cheese. For a hot dip, heat the beans and hummus in a small pan over medium heat, stirring constantly. Add to the bowl, and then layer the ingredients as described above.

LUNCH: MARCONA SALAD

This is adapted from a groovy lunch salad that I stumbled upon in the Carolinas, y'all. Marcona almonds are from Spain and have a buttery, sweet flavor. They're a little more expensive than regular almonds, but their amazing flavor is worth it.

Onto your favorite salad greens, put 1/4 cup of roasted Marcona almonds, a quarter of a grated green apple, thinly sliced red onion, and a crumble of blue cheese. Toss with your favorite balsamic dressing and devour.

DINNER: THE DON'S TUSCAN TOMATO ALL'AGLIONE

Serves 2

I led a culinary coup to get us this recipe. It comes straight from Tuscany and my good friend, cook, and Italy aficionado Don Matteson, aka The Don. He made this at his last dinner party, which he demanded that I attend in order to reveal the dish to me. It was a tough recon job, but hey—I'll do anything for your health.

It's bursting with sweet tomato and garlic flavors infused with fragrant basil, and it is perfecto for a solo plate or to share with guests.

thing, and how I wasn't telling her anything she didn't already know, a claim that one look at her Plank Pose—or her attitude—would tell you wasn't true. The other participants saw her for what she was: someone unable to get past her own expectations.

I'd like to tell you that it all rolled off my duck-like, waterproof yogic back, but truth be told, it really got on my last nerve. I wanted people to like the workshop. I'm a healing practitioner, and I wanted to help her feel better—and I wanted to be invited back again. These desires made me vulnerable to insecurity and anxiety.

I'd already spoken to her and asked her to bring any concerns to me, or the management, so we could try to help her get more out of the program, but she just said no one could help her like something she hated. Fair enough.

I sought out the director of the center and had a frank chat with her over lunch. I expected her to side with the student and tell me to be as compassionate as I could toward her. She leaned forward over her chai, looked left and right, and then whispered, "Congratulations." She said that the most well-known teachers get feedback forms that range from "Best workshop ever—it totally blew my mind" to "I can't stand this awful teacher . . . they're the Devil incarnate."

"At that level," she explained, "there is very little in-between." She counseled me to accept that when you are offering something authentically, there ain't much "meh" but there is a whole lot of love or hate. "You've just gone polar," she said, "and here we see that as a very good sign."

I went back, head held high, and let #30 sip her bamboo thermos full of Haterade while I refocused my attention on doing what I do best: teach. She didn't change, but I did, and it felt great.

On the last day, while everyone else was in their final resting pose, #30 got up and came up to sit on the platform with me. Not the best time or place for a conversation, but I was already past expecting anything else from her. She just wanted to let me know—loudly—that she learned absolutely nothing from me and that she was deeply disappointed in her experience.

I simply said, "Thank you. And—*you're welcome.*" She looked confused, so I explained, "I'm thanking you for being my teacher, one who helped me become even more confident in my message. And you're welcome, because although I don't think you see it this way, this week I showed you where and who you *don't* want to be, and directed you toward your next best path. So in that way, I've been your teacher all along." Her eyes opened wide and filled with tears.

She realized that what I said was another truth she could choose if she wanted to, and to her credit, she did, looking me in the eye, bringing her palms together at her chest, and bowing deeply to me.

This gesture in yoga means *namaste,* which translates to "The light in me honors the light in you, and in that place, we are One," or, as a *Star Wars* fan might say, "May the Force be with you." Then she proceeded to go lie down on her mat and rest with the other students. For the remainder of the last day, she was quiet and, from what I heard, changed her tune about me. But I had ceased to care, because I had done battle with the bitch, both the one reflected outside and the one inside of me that doubted my truth. Now, how does all of this apply to you?

How many times have you been upset because someone treated you poorly or you missed the lesson of learning who you don't want to be when you decided that *this right here* isn't supposed to be happening? Did you fall prey to the illusion that an unpleasant moment was nothing more than a big, stupid, worthless rock standing in the way of all the good stuff you're supposed to be doing? When you think you've missed the party, or you are confronted by an outer bitch (or an inner one in the form of self-criticism and resistance), remember this: nothing happens *to* you . . . only *for* your Core Strength, growth, wisdom, and self-knowledge. If you choose it. Today, we "Bow to the Bitch," wherever we find her, because we yogis know that every #30 has a gift to offer us. People often think that because something—a relationship, a meeting, an event—did not meet their expectations, the time and effort involved was wasted. This kind of experience still holds major value to help you grow and move forward. Everything you don't like points directly to your dharma, or right path, and helps you get out that weed whacker of aligned action to clear it.

So, next time you meet something or someone that rubs you the wrong way, take a deep breath, and instead of losing your cool, smile and say, "Namaste . . . Bitches." Then walk in the other direction.

YOGA

On your mat, it's easy to meet your inner bitch. You do it every time you tell yourself you suck because you didn't get the handstand and everyone else did. Humans are competitive by nature, and that can be healthy fuel to help you progress, but self-criticism is a fantastic way to devalue yourself and diminish your spirit.

It's time to ditch the bitch. To go from snarky to centered, focus on a crucial aspect of every yoga pose—your Earth-to-Core Connection. Remember, what you press down must come up. And the way you come up matters. You'll avoid injury and strain and gain way more lightness and power in each pose when you use gravity to your advantage. Using momentum from the foundation to rocket upward and turbo-charge your core mirrors how you can use every moment to help you fly in your life off the mat, too.

Begin with 3 to 5 rounds of your Core Warm-Up.

Crow

You'll twist, tone the arms, detox, and light up your core line—and then stretch all around your heart center and chest, pulling energy up and spreading the love like your own personal Woodstock. It won't be easy . . . but it will be powerful.

- ☽ Walk your feet together, bend your knees, and roll up into Chair Pose.

- Bow forward, and plant your hands at the front of the mat.

- Press your hands down strongly, middle fingers forward.

- Pull your elbows in toward each other till your forearms are parallel.

- Press your knees into your upper arms, and press your shoulders back out into the arms. Keep your hips low.

- Look gently forward.

- Press your hands into the floor to activate the core: round your back straight up as you slide your elbows forward until they stack directly over your wrists.

- Bring one and maybe both feet in toward the sitting bones.

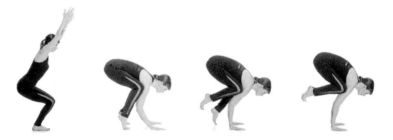

Practice or fly your Crow for 5 breaths! Try to hop off your arms back into Downward-Facing Dog. Take a Vinyasa flow here.

Waterfall Warrior

Bow with humility to your inner strength, and release the inner bitch. You'll counterstretch your Crow, detox your whole body, and strengthen the legs and core more.

FROM DOWNWARD-FACING DOG:

- Inhale to Dog Splits.

- Exhale through Core Plank and step the right foot to the right thumb.

- Inhale, and wave your spine longer.

- Exhale, ground your back foot, and roll up into Warrior I.

- Your hips and back leg spin back a bit to protect the knee as your chest turns forward.

Hold Warrior I for 3 to 5 breaths, noticing that if you don't ground your feet, your pose loses power and gets heavy. Keep rooting down the whole time!

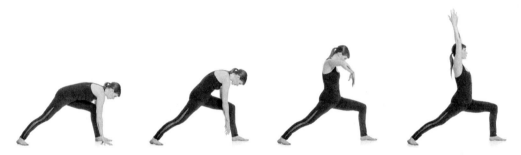

- Inhale, and fly your arms back behind you as you lean forward.

- Exhale, and clasp your hands, palms facing each other.

- Inhale, scoop your front pelvis and spine in and up, and roll up to lift the chest.

- Exhale, fold forward on or inside the front knee.

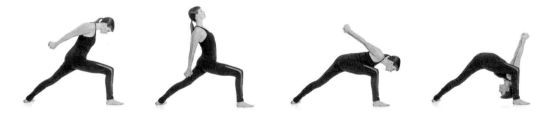

- Inhale, press your feet like mad, lift your toes, and roll back up through your core again to offer the heart to the sky.

  Repeat Waterfall Warrior 3 to 5 times. On your last exhale into your bowing Waterfall Warrior, hold for 3 breaths.

Moonwalk Lunge

Use the warming of Waterfall Warrior to open the hips and release any old fears that led to superbitch behavior. Remember to still ground down through your foundation and keep the hips a little lifted so that you don't strain your joints.

- Lift your back heel, place the knee down, and point the back toes.

- Angle your front right foot open diagonally to the right.

- Roll open your front knee, and come to the pinkie-toe edge of your front foot.

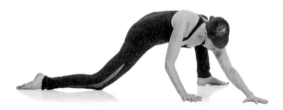

- Walk both hands to the left, chest facing the floor.

- Reach your right hand much longer than the left.

- Inhale to stretch your right side more fully.

Breathe in Moonwalk Lunge for 3 to 5 breaths. Step back to Downward-Facing Dog; Vinyasa if you wish.

Repeat from Crow on the other side. End in Simple Squat or Child's Pose.

When you finish, end with your Core Cooldown.

Namaste! Good job today.

FOOD

Getting enough vegetables into your day can be a real bitch, I know. Eating to fuel your health and satisfy your tastebuds is both an art and a full-time job. Of course it's worth it, but it's also just another thing to carry on your plate, literally. Yet inherently choosing to fuel yourself properly isn't ultimately about food. It's about your self-worth.

To say "yes" to your veggies is to directly confront the inner B who doesn't like herself very much, wants you to eat terribly, and then hates you for it. Enough. It's time for your Core Strength to take the lead and say "no" to punishing yourself with toxic junk.

Whether putting it in your mouth or allowing it to come at you in the form of demeaning relationships, words, or choices, you gain more power and more life force in every way when you decide to act in your own best interests. Today you're going to make that bitch get clean and eat her greens.

RECIPES

BREAKFAST: WILD BACON FRITTATA

You'll be so busy digging the bacon that you won't even notice how healthy this is.

Today, add to your frittata 1 cup of the darkest, wildest, most flavorful greens you have around; 1 strip cooked, chopped bacon; 1 cup of any leftover veggies, sliced thin.

SNACK

Have a fruit-and-yogurt parfait of your creation today as a sweet, creamy treat between two veggie-heavy meals.

LUNCH: GREEN MACHINE SMOOTHIE

Serves 1 to 2

It's a full-on salad in a glass, which sounds kind of awful, until you taste it.

1 banana, frozen and halved

1 cup spinach

half an avocado, pitted

1 scoop Vega One Vanilla Chai mix
  or protein powder

1 cup coconut or almond milk

1/4 teaspoon cinnamon

1 tablespoon coconut oil

Put all items in a blender, and blend on High, then Medium, then High again to pulverize all the spinach.

DINNER: ZAMAS' LIME-GARLIC FISH DISH

Serves 2

While I was in Tulum, Mexico, writing this book, I came across Zamas, a beautiful beachfront restaurant. I was lured there by the sounds of a local guitarist, but I stayed for one of the best fish dishes I've ever had. Daniel, the owner, was kind enough to share the recipe with us.

1 cup grain of choice

sprinkle of sea salt

dash of red pepper flakes

1 to 2 large cloves garlic

1/2 cup fresh lime or lemon juice

1/2 cup water

2 (6-ounce) white fish fillets, like halibut
  or tilapia

salt and pepper to taste

2 cups fresh spinach or arugula

sliced lime or lemon, for garnish

Prepare your grain on the stove or in a rice cooker with the necessary water, add salt and red pepper flakes for heat. When finished, keep covered until the fish is done.

Place the garlic, lime or lemon juice, and water in a blender and puree. Set aside. Either grill the fish or cook in a lightly oiled, hot pan. Season the fish with salt and pepper, and drizzle half of the citrus/garlic sauce onto the fish as it cooks. Save the rest.

On a plate, layer the cooked grain, then the greens, and then the fish on top to wilt the greens. Top with the rest of your citrus sauce to taste, and garnish with a lime or lemon slice and a light dusting of red pepper flakes.

BEVERAGES: CUCUMBER/LEMON/MINT-INFUSED WATER

I think drinking water is as boring as watching paint dry. Yet we must. That's why I always have a big glass jug of filtered water infused with something or other sitting in the fridge. It makes me happy to look at the beautiful concoction and inspires me to drink more.

    1 cucumber, peeled and sliced

    1/2 cup fresh mint leaves

    2 lemons, sliced

Put all the ingredients into a covered glass pitcher or jar. Fill with filtered water, and let sit in the fridge overnight if possible. Pour water through a strainer before drinking. Enjoy!

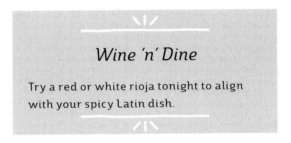

Wine 'n' Dine

Try a red or white rioja tonight to align with your spicy Latin dish.

ACTION: SNARKY LITTLE BITCH (SLB) AND THE TIMES THREE TECHNIQUE

It's not cute to be a Snarky Little Bitch (SLB). Although you might get a fleeting, faux-powerful feeling—and even a laugh when you belittle or judge others—those around you will know deep down that when the tables are turned, you'll criticize them, too, behind their backs. Not exactly a way to win friends or trust.

What we practice, we get better at, whether it's containing our anger or expressing it, doing a Crow pose, moving toward health or away—or being a Snarky Little Bitch. Today, I invite you to try this zippy little negative-energy-clearing technique.

The Times Three Technique: Whenever you catch yourself being an SLB toward yourself or others (Ex: "OMG. Look at her butt. It's so big. Glad I work out.")...

immediately counteract by saying or thinking something positive—*that you actually believe*—three times (Ex: "Girlfriend, rock that juicy booty!").

This seemingly simple switch actually is quite powerful. Like any repetitive thought or habit, it rewires your brain so that you pave superhighways to your integrity. After a while, you'll become much less inclined toward Snarky Little Bitch behavior, because you'll have practiced being the kinder, gentler you three times more often.

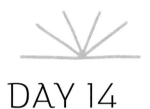

DAY 14

THEME: Eyewitness

My life is hectic. So when I need to gain some perspective, I step back from my routine and get away ... far, far away. Now, when you think of a vacation, you probably imagine sun, frolicking by the water, and lounging with a mango margarita in hand while soaking up the rays. So do I. I've tried a few places on for size, but the one that fits me the best so far is Tulum, on the east coast of Mexico; however, last time I was there, I got a hurricane instead of a sunny paradise.

One morning I was on a beach walk under a clear blue sky when I turned around to head back to the resort center. Over the ocean, blocking out all sunlight, was a pure black wall of hell's fury barreling toward shore—right toward *me*, in fact. I stuck my iPod under my arm and did the only thing I could think of: I ran.

Within about five minutes, what began as a steady but manageable rainstorm turned into a vortex that hit me like the last round in *Rocky IV*. It was hard to run forward, and at some points, I truly felt lifted off the sand. I could have freaked out and let the storm make it all the way inside my mind and heart, but I was stubbornly focused on my goal to see myself unharmed, wrapped in a towel, with a mango margarita in my hand. I chose to embrace the heightening of sensation instead of letting it take me down into the abyss of anxiety and fear.

Yogis know how to move fast on the outside but keep calm within. I finally made it to the restaurant of my beachfront hotel, where the staff helpfully got me that towel and margarita and, not so helpfully, took a photo of my raccoon eyes (yes, I put on mascara for my walk) and, I have a sneaking suspicion, posted it to Facebook. Then I busted out my computer and journal, and spent the rest of the trip—four more days, ensconced cozily in my cabana or the lounge, writing, while Mother Nature had her way with the beach.

And you know what? It was one of the best trips of my life. Because it was the off-season, I was the only guest. I wasn't there to meet a man, entertain others, or be entertained. What I needed, and what I got, was solitude and a time to re-center, listen inside, and auto-tune with nature just by being so close to her in all her many moods.

Today, you'll learn to weather any inner or outer storm as you face the unpredictable winds of change *and* still stand strong at the calm center. When you become even more skilled at existing in these two places at once, then you're well on your way to gaining the elusive calm so many people seek—not only after the emotional hurricanes that will surely come your way but *during* them, as well.

YOGA

Many people can stay in equilibrium just fine when life is sunny, but when the proverbial sh*t hits the fan, they lose it faster than fat around Jillian Michaels.

Yoga can teach you to access your best ally against unmooring from your core: the Witness, that neutral observer status you can employ regardless of what other people, places, or things decide to throw at you. Today you'll literally get more grounded with moves I designed to help you experience and, over time, master your ability to feel strong sensations and still act from, and with, assured integrity.

When you do each pose today, focus on your breathing, and see if you can stay aware of what's happening, without naming it as good or bad, or judging yourself. A dedication to feel intensity and at the same time to step back, relax, refuse to take anything personally, and witness your moment is all it takes.

Today I invite you to put your knees down in Lunges, Plank, and

Chaturanga. Do less in your poses, and make it more of an earth-to-core practice.

Begin with 3 to 5 rounds of your Core Warm-Up.

FLOW 1: LOW WARRIOR FLOW

These warrior variations will ground and open you in new ways, and allow you to feel these poses more than endure them. Let your breath move, and become more aware of the constant wave upward from earth to your belly, pelvis, and low back in each moment. The true Warrior forces nothing and allows everything to naturally unfold.

Put a folded blanket or soft towel under your back knee for padding.

Repeat each of the following poses for 5 to 10 breaths or repetitions each.

Hands and Knees Core Plank

- Come onto your hands and knees.

- Inhale, and lift your left leg up behind you.

- Exhale, bend knee into chest, and round your back.

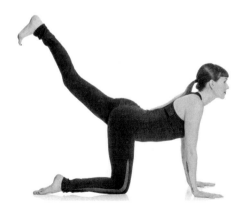
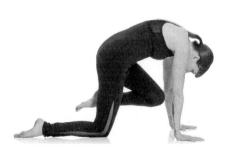

Knee-Down Low Lunge

✣ On your last exhale, step your right foot to the right thumb. Your left shin is parallel to the left long edge of your mat, foot pointed.

✣ Exhale, roll up into Low Lunge, and reach your arms into the air.

✣ Draw your top front pelvic bones in and up, even as you lean forward gently into the hip stretch.

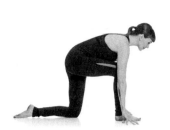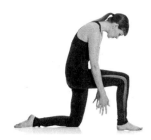

Cat/Cow Low Lunge

✣ Plant your palms on your front thigh.

✣ Inhale, and arch your spine.

✣ Exhale, and round in, chin toward chest.

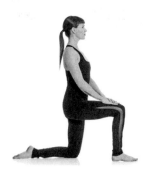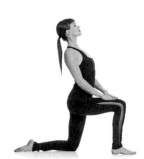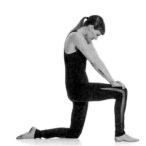

Low Warrior 1 to Low Waterfall Warrior

✣ Angle your back shin and foot diagonally so that the foot points at the back right corner of your mat.

✣ Reach arms up from here.

- Interlace your fingers, palms facing each other.

- Inhale, roll back up, and lift your lower belly and your chest.

- Exhale, and pour your body over your front thigh or inside it for Low Waterfall Warrior.

- Inhale, and roll back up, hands still clasped.

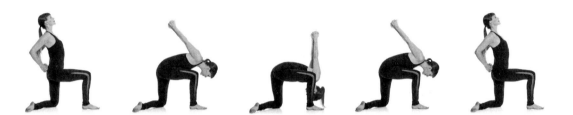

Repeat Waterfall Warrior for 3 to 5 breaths; then hold your last folded exhale for 3 to 5 breaths. Locate your witness, and observe the sensations you feel as you maintain a rhythmic Golden Flame breath.

After Waterfall Warrior, fold back into Child's Pose for one minute or so. Then return to hands and knees, and repeat the entire sequence on the other side.

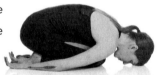

Yin Goddess

After your last Waterfall Warrior, take Goddess Pose lying on your back today, but do it Yin-style. This is a longer hold, so totally relax your muscles, to give a slight stimulating tug on the connective tissue around the joints instead of the stretch you associate with muscles. Completely relax in a position where you feel a light stretch somewhere in the hips, groins, lower back, and spine.

Find the center of any storm of sensation as you release, reflect, and breathe for 3 to 5 minutes in the pose.

When you finish, end with your Core Cooldown.

Namaste! Good job today.

FOOD

Inflammation is one of the biggest firestorms you can create inside your body. It ain't pretty: even one day of inflammatory response speeds up your aging process, creates bloat, puts your immune system into overdrive, exhausts you, and is a precursor to most every major disease. One way we trigger this storm is by eating foods that fuel inflammation instead of energy. To calm this storm, choose your food wisely.

This requires you to become an eyewitness as you take a nonjudgmental look at what you have been eating until now. Many of our grocery stores are full of GMO, processed, chemical-filled products, some of which look like real food but are firebombs disguised as nutrition. I mean... "cheese *food*"? What is *that*? Today we clear out the foods that cause imbalances and replace them with life-enhancing, firefighting foods to help you maintain your cool both inside and out.

RECIPES

BREAKFAST: BLACK-AND-BLUE SMOOTHIE

Fruits (organic) of all kinds punch inflammation right in the kisser. So make your first meal a cooling knockout! Today add blueberries, blackberries, and half a cucumber to your mix.

SNACK: APPLE PIE YOGURT

This chillaxing addition to yogurt, quinoa, cereal, or toast is chock-full of fiber and protein but tastes like apple-pie filling. Bonus!

1 apple, cored and diced, peeled or not	1 tablespoon chopped nuts
big sprinkle of cinnamon	honey to taste
	dash of olive oil

Sauté the apples, cinnamon, chopped nuts, and honey in a hot pan with a little olive oil until the apples become soft. Cool in a dish in the fridge for 10 minutes before serving.

LUNCH: SAVORY-SWEET SKILLET SALAD

This is a cornucopia of anti-inflammatory foods. Eat this dish for more energy and to quench any fires that are burning you out. Today, make your skillet salad, and add some or all of the following: half a portobello mushroom, sliced thick; 1 cup sugar snap peas or a handful of spinach or arugula; 1/2 red bell pepper, de-seeded and sliced; 1 garlic clove, diced; 1/8 red onion, sliced thin; dressing of choice.

DINNER: SALMON WITH COOLING EDAMAME COCONUT RICE

Serves 2

Your rice is going to steal the show; if you don't keep an eye on it your guest will eat it all. Edamame (soybeans) are one of the only vegetables with all the amino acids you need to make a complete protein. If tofu or soy protein powder upsets your stomach, edamame might work better for your belly. The omegas in salmon are powerful inflammation fighters, too.

1 cup brown rice	1 tablespoon raisins
1/2 cup coconut milk	1 tablespoon olive oil
1/2 cup water	2 (6-ounce) salmon fillets
1/2 cup shelled edamame, fresh, canned, or frozen	dash of sea salt, pepper
1 tablespoon cashews, whole or chopped	2 thin lime slices

Place the rice, coconut milk, water, and edamame in a rice cooker or saucepan. Cook until there are 5 minutes left; then add the nuts and raisins. Stir once, and cook until done. Cook the salmon in a medium-hot pan with olive oil, sea salt, and pepper until cooked to your desired doneness. Place a portion of the rice mixture on each plate, and top with salmon. Garnish with lime slices and serve.

BEVERAGES: AWESOME ALMOND MILK

P.S. I got both of these recipes from my rocker vegan friend Paul Jarvis, who wrote an ebook called *Eat Awesome*.

Homemade almond milk is delicious and easy to make at home. Use it anywhere you'd use the regular stuff. It's easier than you think, and to sweeten the deal, if you make the milk, you can have cheesecake. Yup! Cheesecake (see below).

1 cup unsalted, raw almonds

3 1/2 cups water

2 pitted dates or 2 teaspoons maple syrup

few drops vanilla extract

dash of cinnamon

Soak almonds in water for 1 hour. Discard soaking water. Rinse almonds and place in a blender with water and dates if you're using them. Puree thoroughly. Drape cheese-cloth or a very thin dish towel over a large bowl. (If you're going to make this a lot, buy a nut sack expressly for this purpose. Yes, it's called a nut sack. I know, I know. . . . You can find them at most health food stores.)

Pour the mixture into the towel, and gather the corners up so that you can squeeze and strain the liquid through into the bowl. Add the vanilla, cinnamon, and maple syrup, if using, to the liquid. Rinse the blender, pour the liquid back into the blender, and blend again on Low for a few seconds. Reserve the nut meal (the leftover from your squeeze) in a medium bowl for your dessert. Refrigerate or freeze the meal if you're not using it today.

Put the milk into a sealed glass jar or pitcher in the fridge. Keeps for 2 to 4 days.

Use the almond milk in your tea or coffee today, and ice it for a cooling drink.

DESSERT: RAWESOME CHEESECAKE

I couldn't believe how good this pie tasted—and how good it was for me. I think you'll love it, and you'll never miss the dairy.

2 cups cashews

3/4 cup pitted dates

1 cup almond meal

juice of 2 lemons

2 teaspoons maple syrup

1 cup berries, fresh or frozen

Soak the cashews in a bowl of water for 1 hour. In a blender, roughly blend the dates together with the almond meal until smooth but not pureed. Press this mixture into an 8-inch pie pan to make the crust. Rinse the blender, and puree the cashews, lemon juice, and maple syrup. Ladle this filling on top of the crust evenly. Cover and freeze for an hour.

Puree the berries in the blender until smooth. Store, covered, in the refrigerator to cool.

Defrost the pie in the fridge for about an hour; then cut and serve. It should be cold enough to hold together in slices but not frozen. Drizzle the pureed fruit on top of each slice. Serve.

ACTION: THUNDERSTORM MEDITATION

This technique helps you create a calm oasis in your mind, no matter what the mental weather.

I use it anytime I feel stress rising. In two minutes, you too can come back to a freakin' fabulously peaceful place instead of being pelted by your thoughts all night like a grade school game of dodgeball.

Get your Zs, dissolve anxiety, and relax . . . it's all found here in the eye of the storm:

- Come to a sitting position or lie down.

- Begin to slow your breath through the nose (use the Double-Down Breath Technique if you want).

- Close your eyes, and envision you're in a really comfy place with some kind of a force field or wall, like a cozy bed with a nice comforter and pillows, and maybe by a fireplace in a nice room. Sometimes I think of being on a beach enclosed in a huge hamster exercise ball. I know, I'm weird. (Anyway, pick your best vision.)

- Imagine that your thoughts are made of raindrops. They can be in the shape of actual words or images or just big blobs of rain.

- Focus your attention on how satisfied and safe, and even sleepy, you are, right where you are.

∗ Notice that all thoughts, and I mean all, are unable to get to your happy place, because as they hit the protective boundary you've created, they splash into it and harmlessly run down the outside like the rainwater they are.

∗ If your thoughts start creeping in again, realize that you are much stronger than they are. You're their master, not their victim. Gently turn your attention back to not allowing them in, as easy as a gentle summer rain.

The more you practice this, the more habitual the visualization will become and the faster you'll find yourself in your sleepy sweet spot. I slip into this most nights now without even thinking, and it's also perfect for a quick detachment from any sticky, anxious thoughts that arise during the day.

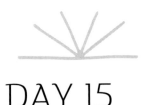

DAY 15

THEME: DIFY

Last night I was sitting in one of my favorite restaurants, a French/ Mexican place in Brooklyn. It was packed, as tends to happen at 8 p.m. on a Friday night around here. I saw five girls gussied up for a night out walk up to the French host and ask him the standard question: "How long for a table?"

Now, during the evening rush, the standard response is "twenty minutes" regardless of whether or not there's an ice cube's chance in hell that you'll be sitting down anytime within the next hour. The host looks at the women, raises his eyebrow Frenchily, and gestures over at all the tables full of people happily munching away and talking: "Look at zem all, eating. Zey are right in ze meeddle of zeir meals. I could tell you twenty meenutes, but what can I do? Zey could be an hour, two hours, who can say? I cannot rush zeir pleasure."

Now that's a host, there to protect pleasure, not please. Needless to say, the girls were not happy. They wanted to hear twenty minutes, even if it wasn't true. So they got miffed and stormed out. The host looked at me, shrugged his shoulders, and then turned right back to his post. I got goose bumps. Because, *exactly*: What, ultimately, can any of us do if we want to represent our core truths out into the world? Lie? Hide? Or say clearly, unapologetically what we mean. I don't think it serves anyone when we choose to placate others and not risk ruffling feathers over being real.

In the end, life is a DIFY (do it for yourself) project. I'm not asking you to discount everyone else's needs and feelings or to be rude. I *am* inviting you to take your truth into account just a little more, express it when asked, and make sure you're living authentically as yourself instead of wearing the costume of the person you think makes everyone like you.

This is challenging for many people. I hear it all the time: "I'm afraid that if I speak up or demand change, he/she will leave me." "I don't have the money to get a job I like, so I have to stay in this one that stresses me out." "I don't want to disappoint or confront people, so I keep my opinions to myself."

Today this stops. Say your truth is that your job isn't right for you. Your boss may not like it, and your partner may freak out about the perceived lack of stability. You will have to expend some effort to look for new work or create an additional income stream that allows you to leave. You might feel afraid, unsure, or alone. But guess what? Living from your truth means that you deeply respect not only yourself but also those in your life.

You are now going to be brave, be genuine, reclaim reality, and give others all the information they need to decide if they can live their best truth around you instead of keeping them in the dark so that they won't get upset, confront you, or leave you. That's not love talking, that's fear.

Living authentically requires you to endure the discomfort of people not getting behind or liking your choices, because they think they know what's best for you. Yet courage attracts courage. This is what it looks and feels like to truly honor yourself, invest in your own good time, and welcome those whose truths resonate with yours to join the party.

Pour all your energy not into convincing those who cannot be convinced or letting fear win, but into leading your best life by example. Today you begin your biggest DIFY job ever: excavating your truth and renovating your life from the inside out. Vive la Révolution!

YOGA

So, how do we put this concept of DIFY into action on the mat? When it comes to moving through life and yoga, watch the times when you try to wear the mask of who you think you should be physically, mentally, or spiritually. Are you acting "yogier-than-thou"? Have you become an evangelical yogi or yogini, espousing doctrine and criticizing others who don't share your beliefs or singular "way" of practicing? Do you try to force an advanced pose when your lower back is screaming at you?

As you've learned by now, this is not the Yoga Body way. Instead, *do your practice for yourself.* Even as you stretch your arms and legs outward, make the interior alignment of your sacrum and lower-back spine a priority. It is the core area that takes so much abuse in our daily lives that it needs an infusion of constant spaciousness and support.

Above all, approach your poses with an intention to remain bona fide and you'll honestly shine, no matter how straight your legs get today.

Begin with 5 rounds of your Core Warm-Up so that you're nice and heated for today's sequences!

HALF-BIND FLOW

Today is the start of your Expression week, so you'll start working into more extremity-opening postures. See if you can get down and dedicated enough to hold fast to your pelvic and spinal alignment.

Half-Bound Half-Moon Pose

⁖ Come into Downward-Facing Dog.

⁖ Exhale your left foot to the left thumb.

- Inhale, wave your spine longer.

- Exhale, roll up into Warrior II.

- Step the back foot forward halfway up your mat.

- Reach your left hand forward to the ground on Spidey fingertips placed wide of the left shoulder.

- Root your left foot into the floor, and lift power through the leg, beginning to straighten it, as you center the pelvis and lower back in and up from both front and back.

- Unfurl the right hip and arm open to the sky, keeping the right leg parallel to the mat.

- Internally rotate your top arm so that the palm faces behind you. Plug your shoulder and armpit back to align the shoulder joint.

- Half-bind: bend your raised arm so that the back of your hand is on your back. Your hand may even come all the way around, fingers into your left hip crease.

- The more your top hip opens, the more the front leg externally rotates to keep facing forward.

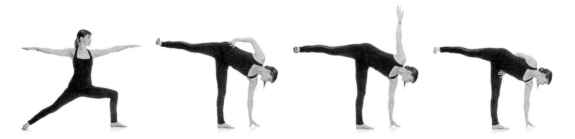

Take 5 breaths here.

Half-Bound Warrior II

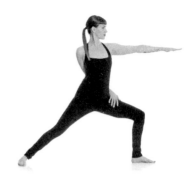

- Keep the top arm bound, and bend your front knee.

- Step mindfully back to ground your back foot down into a Warrior stance.

- Exhale, and roll in and up to a Warrior II position with the back arm bound; the left arm points forward as usual.

Half-Bound Reverse Warrior

As you move through this next flow, be aware of your pelvis's tendency to tilt too far forward or back.

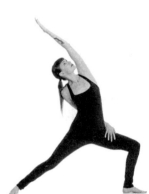

- Inhale, and stretch the spine and left arm in a side bend over the back leg; the right arm is still bound.

Full-Bound Side Angle

- Exhale and place your left forearm onto your left thigh for Half-Bound Side Angle, or round your back down and thread your left arm inside of and under your left thigh.

- Pause here and internally rotate your bottom arm so that the palm faces the sky. Root the shoulder back.

- Bend elbows, and clasp on to your left fingertips or wrist. Straighten your arms more.

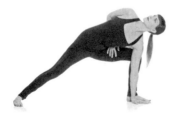 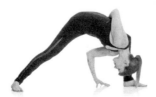 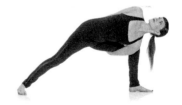

Take 3 breaths here.

Bound Triangle to Triangle Pose

- Lengthen your front leg toward straight, if desired, and then roll the right side of your chest open.

- Reach your bottom hand to the floor outside the leg or onto your shin or block. Finally, unbind the right arm for fully open Triangle Pose. The arm should float up now.

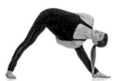 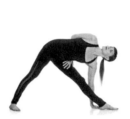 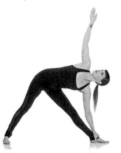

When you finish, find your way into Downward-Facing Dog.

Repeat the sequence on your other side.

End with your Core Cooldown.

Namaste! Good job DIFY-ing today.

FOOD

Not only will you cook for yourself today but you will cook for yourself like a French lovaaah would make your meals: with unapologetic *plaisir.*

Pretend you're in a romantic bistro that only locals know on some cobblestone backstreet, and you're seated at a candlelit table with a quaint checkered tablecloth. Prepare your dishes with gusto; sing, dance, listen to music, and when you eat, enjoy every bite as much as you enjoy being alive, right now in this most *incroyable* moment. Ready? *Allez!*

RECIPES

BREAKFAST: HERBES DE PROVENCE MINIQUICHES

Makes 6 quiches

This recipe turns the oven (or toaster oven) into your friend. I make this dish in a muffin pan. If you don't have one, do this as a regular frittata instead.

olive oil

6 eggs

splash of plain, unsweetened coconut or almond milk

sprinkle of Herbes de Provence (if you, like me, don't like the taste of lavender, substitute finely chopped chives, basil, or rosemary instead)

sea salt and freshly ground black pepper

2 handfuls fresh chopped spinach

1/2 cup chopped cooked regular, veggie, or turkey bacon

grated Parmesan

1 medium-size potato, grated and fried (see below)

6 thin slices tomato (optional)

Preheat the oven to 375°F. Wipe the muffin tins with a light coat of olive oil.

Whisk the eggs, milk, and Herbes de Provence together in a bowl. Add salt and pepper to taste. Stir in the rest of the ingredients except the tomato.

Fill each muffin cup almost to the top with the egg mixture. I like to add a slice of tomato to the top of each one for dramatic effect (so very French).

Bake until the mixture is set in the center, about 8 to 10 minutes.

Optional: If you have time, grate the potato into a hot, olive-oiled pan, and stir until browned. Add to the egg mix for a crispy surprise in each quiche. Serve warm and/or refrigerate for later.

LUNCH: NIÇOISE SALAD AU-VOCADO

This is a great take on the classic Niçoise. If you're particularly hungry, add the avocado and tuna mix to your usual salad.

1 can albacore, dolphin-free tuna (packed in water)

1 teaspoon balsamic vinegar

1 scallion, minced

1/4 red bell pepper, seeded and finely chopped

salt and pepper to taste

2 teaspoons olive oil

1/2 avocado, pitted

In a small bowl, mix together all the ingredients except for the avocado. In the place where the avocado pit was, place a heaping mound of your tuna mix. Eat with a spoon or dipping chips, and add more tuna if needed as you go.

SNACK: COCONUT MOCHA

You had such a protein-packed salad for lunch that your blood sugar is chillin' like Bob Dylan. Let's bridge meals with a sweet treat that's très healthy, though you'd never know. It reminds me of many a breakfast in France, where pain au chocolat is a staple. Make this with or without the coffee, as you wish.

1 (4-ounce) cup coffee or
   1 teaspoon instant coffee

1 cup coconut milk

1 tablespoon cocoa powder

agave nectar to taste

cinnamon, for garnish

In a pan, heat and whisk the coconut milk and cocoa powder. Add the agave to taste. Pour the milk mixture over the half a cup of coffee, or add the instant coffee right into the milk mixture. Garnish with a sprinkle of cinnamon and serve.

DINNER: SAUTÉED SHRIMP WITH PROVENÇALE SAUCE

Serves 2

This simple, fragrant, and savory topping takes any protein and turns it up to 11. It's so good I'd eat it on a shoe. A Louboutin, but still.

FOR THE PROVENÇALE SAUCE

1/2 cup olive oil

1/3 cup finely chopped onions

1 cup diced fresh tomato

1/2 clove garlic, minced

1 teaspoon Herbes de Provence
   (or just add some chopped
   rosemary and sage)

2 cups tomato sauce

1 tablespoon capers

1 tablespoon chopped Kalamata olives

sea salt to taste

freshly ground black pepper to taste

FOR THE SHRIMP

Olive oil

12 ounces organic fresh or frozen shrimp

2 cloves garlic, sliced

4 cups whole green beans, tips removed

For the sauce

In a heavy-bottomed saucepan, sauté the onions in the heated olive oil until they're translucent, about 5 minutes.

Add the tomato, garlic, and Herbes de Provence. Continue to sauté until the tomatoes are soft, about 10 minutes.

Add the tomato sauce, capers, olives, salt, and pepper, and bring to a simmer. Reduce for about 10 minutes. Set aside.

Wine 'n' Dine

Pair this dish with a fresh red wine like a Beaujolais Nouveau or a more earthy Saint-Émilion.

For the shrimp

In a medium-hot pan coated with olive oil, sauté the shrimp until cooked through, 2 to 3 minutes per side. Do not overcook. Divide the shrimp between two plates.

In another pan, heat olive oil over medium heat. Cook the garlic till golden, add the green beans, and cook to your desired doneness.

Spoon the sauce over the shrimp, and divide the beans between the two plates. I like to serve this with a side of sea-salted and lime-spritzed quinoa.

DESSERT: AVOCADO DARK CHOCOLATE MOUSSE

Serves 2

This is one of those healthy things that sounds utterly disgusting until you taste it. Then you'll be the one trying to convince people to just . . . take . . . one . . . bite. Welcome to my world.

1 ripe avocado, peeled and pitted

2 tablespoons cocoa powder, plus more for sprinkling

2 tablespoons agave nectar

½ tablespoon vanilla extract

pinch of cinnamon

good pinch chipotle powder or cayenne pepper (if you want a kick)

Place all the ingredients in a blender and blend, scraping the sides of the blender and alternating between High and Low for 2 to 3 minutes until smooth. Serve in a pretty glass or bowl with a sprinkle of cocoa and cinnamon on top.

ACTION: SELF-CENTERING SEVEN

Do tell: what top seven (or more) aspects of a person's character do you require in order to let them into your most intimate circle?

Some that my clients commonly expect in a mate or close friend are

- honesty, authenticity

- loyalty, faithfulness

- doing their own work, creatively, mentally, emotionally

- sense of humor, ability to lighten up and see the positive

- supportive and understanding

- forgiving of others' mistakes and their own

- unconditionally loving

Now, turn this right back around on yourself. Are you exhibiting these same qualities toward yourself and the people you say you care about? Do you want people to tell you things they don't mean and not show you who they are? Of course not. You want to know where you stand with them. It's a gift that you give yourself and those in your life, and, ultimately, that gift is freedom—freedom *to* be yourself and freedom *from* the constriction of being any less than that, ever.

Today, begin lovingly but clearly speaking and acting from your truth even more. If you want some alone time instead of going out, take it. If someone asks you if you liked a movie you know they loved, don't say you loved it too for their sake. Tell them what you really think; otherwise, you're going to have to give that lie CPR whenever they're around.

Even little white lies end up being a smoke screen over your true nature that eat away at the foundation of your confidence and Core Strength. Enough of these and your foundation will crumble. Shore it up, starting now.

You might be surprised to learn that most people already know where you have been acting, and though they may not agree with your more truthful take, they will usually respect you much more for speaking your mind and heart.

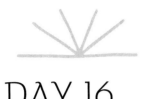

DAY 16

THEME: Get a Tattoo

Today bit the big one. It was so bad that *one of those days* was having one of those days. It didn't start out that way, though. I got up early, feeling just a little bit taller, shooting creative energy hoops like a baller, excited to go to the café and write another, much more uplifting chapter than this one.

My favorite coffee shop is a twenty-minute walk, and I pack for it like a Nepalese Sherpa. 'Cause ain't no tellin' when I'm going home again. This distance is not so great if, say, one forgets all one's money and credit cards in one's other purse and only realizes it after slogging all the way there in 93-degree heat, ordering a drink, and hearing the girl behind the counter say, "That'll be $3.95," while there are five people in line impatiently waiting. So I walked all the way back home. Got the money. Then back to the café. Note to Self: Sadie, your black Frye motorcycle boots are hot. In a *shin-sauna kind of* way. Buy some sandals.

I finally arrive back at the coffee shop, paid for my drink, got all settled at a table with my chai, and, before I could take a sip, proceeded to knock it all over the table and computer. I miraculously saved the computer from saturation, cleaned up the table, my lap, and one leg of the guy sitting next to me. I turned on the computer, only to realize simultaneously that I left my power cord at home, and the battery was in the red.

I got online for exactly seven minutes, just enough time for me to see the link sent by my friend that took me to a website with a post dedicated to showing photos of me with arrows pointing out all my physical flaws. Although it stung, I *was* psyched to see that one person in this world thinks I have "too much" junk in my trunk.

My next appointment on this now completely ass-picious day was to get a tattoo. Now, even on the best of days, experiencing a tattoo is about as fun as stubbing your toe repeatedly for an hour straight.

I'd like to tell you that I took my own advice, applied my super-yogi skills, and became the Buddha instead of a harried, twitching, DEFCON-rising ball of irritation. But I can't.

By the time I laid on that table to undergo a needling session, I was down to the last inch of my last rope. So guess what I did to that lucky tattoo artist lady when she started working? I surrendered. I know! It surprised me, too. The moment I felt that crazy, ouchy feeling on my arm, I began to switch my breath deeper. I relaxed my whole body and emotionally *leaned into* the feeling, instead of resisting it.

I ultimately remembered to practice what I wanted to tell you today: that even when we undergo pain—whether physical, emotional, or mental—we don't have to suffer. Life is an alteration of the neutral, the seemingly good, the bad, and the ugly. We all cycle through these states as long as we live. Yet suffering—and its accompanying minions: negative stress, anxiety, depression, and fear—is not something that has to happen to you, at least, not for long. Suffering occurs when you resist what *is*. Most people skip this and go right to wishing that they had *less* or *more* right now.

For example, you might want fewer bills, more attention from your partner, more money, a different job—until your whole life is wasted on wanting something else and waiting instead of living. Now, this doesn't mean that you shouldn't want things to change. This whole book is about doing just that. It means that if you want to cease suffering, even in times of challenge or pain, you must first accept the situation for what it is. Then, once you surrender to reality, you can act from a place of clear-seeing fierceness, not fear.

Acting before acceptance is a bad idea. Any action will come from resistance and is more likely to produce an outcome that perpetuates that resistance. Accepting the existence of your experience is not the same as agreeing with it. Did I like that demeaning website? No. Would I start one just like it? No. Do I accept that it exists and that my feelings around it are real and that I'm bothered by it? Yes.

Did getting the tattoo feel good? No, but by accepting that the reality of getting a tattoo is that it hurts, the pain became simply a sensation. The rest of my day was great, even though other challenges arose, because I remembered how to hug them, take on any lessons that arose, then send them on their way, and not let them get to me. Today you'll learn how to surrender, too, and realize that no matter what tries to poke and sting your heart, body, or mind, it is just a feeling, not your master.

YOGA

Most people are as repelled by discomfort as I am by spending my precious time watching bleached-blond housewives fighting over boob jobs on national TV, and they avoid it at all costs.

So much of what you do is driven by a primordial desire for comfort. In our animal brains, we are all lounge lizards, just big babies who want our blankie back. But get too rolled up in that gooshy burrito of a life-comforter and pretty soon you're not enjoying that downy goodness anymore—you're trapped in it. Transformation is not the same thing as feeling happy all the time. Love, victory, success, breakthrough—all these come at the cost of comfort. You have to pay to play, feel to get real.

Today my invitation to you is simple: invite sensation. Whenever you would usually get the heck out of Dodge in a pose, take at least 1 to 3 more breaths.

Begin with 3 to 5 rounds of your Core Warm-Up.

FLOW 1: FRONT BODY FLOW

It's not only things you don't want that can be intense but also the things you do want, like intimacy, vulnerability, self-knowledge, and love. This flow will open your whole front body and stabilize deep core muscles, balancing your openess to this moment with a strong center.

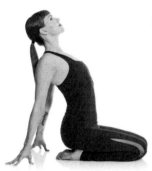

Seated Tabletop

⁘ From Child's Pose, come up to sit on your shins, and walk your fingertips behind your hips.

⁘ Draw the lower belly in and up even as you arch your chest higher, shoulders drawn back.

Waterfall Cobra

⁘ Walk your hands forward toward the front of your mat, and snake onto your belly for Cobra preparation, forehead to the floor.

⁘ Hands plant beside your low ribs, elbows stacked over your wrists.

⁘ Inhale, and prepare. Tuck your tailbone long.

⁘ Exhale, press hands down, and activate your psoas support by rolling up along your front spine as you lift your chest and shoulders into Baby or higher to Teenage Cobra.

⁘ Slide your ears back and up to take the head back with a long spine.

⁘ Exhale, and roll back onto the belly and forehead.

❖ Inhale, roll up again.

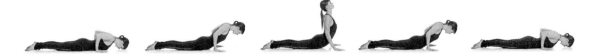

Repeat Waterfall Cobra 3 to 5 times.

Hold your final backbend for 3 to 5 breaths. Come through Child's Pose and stretch into Seated Tabletop again.

Kneeling Plank

❖ From Seated Tabletop, come up to kneel on the mat or a blanket if your knees are sensitive.

❖ Point your toes. Press toenails into the floor.

❖ Draw your top, front pelvic crests and front spine in and up, tailbone long to counterbalance the tendency of the next two poses to cause too much lumbar arching.

❖ Bring your hands to your chest, palms together.

❖ Inhale, and lean back a few inches until your core and thighs engage.

❖ Exhale, and come forward over your knees again.

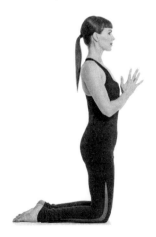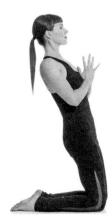

Repeat Kneeling Plank no more than 10 times; more than this can cause uncool soreness.

Fold forward into Child's Pose for 5 to 10 breaths, gently rocking the hips from side to side to release the back muscles.

Camel Pose

∴• Roll back up to kneeling again.

∴• Place your hands on your hips for support.

∴• Inhale, lower your seat toward your heels, and pull up through your inner thighs until your sitting bones open wider behind you. I call this Bootyasana for obvious reasons.

∴• Draw your front pelvis and belly inward to roll up along the front of your spine until you're fully kneeling, hips and thighs stacked over knees.

∴• Your shoulders roll back and shoulder blades lift the back of your heart as if there's a helping hand there.

∴• Slide the ears back and up until you are looking diagonally upward (at the crease between the wall and the ceiling). Do not drop your head back—this can cause spinal compression and artery strain. Yuckasana!

∴• Move right into Camel Circle.

CAMEL CIRCLE

∴• Inhale, and lift your left arm into the air.

∴• Exhale, circle it back, stretch it slowly as you go, and then bring the hand onto the hip again.

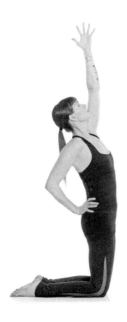
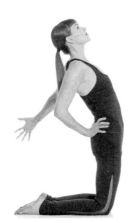

⁖ Switch sides.

Repeat Camel Circle 1 to 3 times on each side.

Fold into Child's Pose for a few moments, and then do one more Camel Circle. Try Full Camel if you can.

FULL CAMEL

⁖ Flex your feet so heels are higher.

⁖ When you lower your hips to your heels, instead of placing your hands on your hips, try grabbing your heels with your palms. Thumbs are on the inside of your ankles, fingers on the outside.

⁖ Roll up through your arms for a deeper backbend.

⁖ Keep your tailbone long and your front spine in and up.

⁖ Try Camel with pointed feet for a deeper backbend.

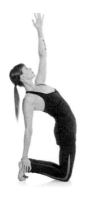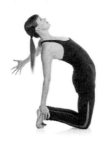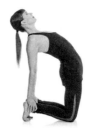

Take 3 to 5 breaths in Full Camel.

Rest in Child's Pose for 1 minute.

End with your Core Cooldown.

Namaste! Good job today.

FOOD

Let's add flavor and heat today—a tattoo for your tongue. I'm not asking you to douse everything with habañero hot sauce until your teeth itch, but wherever your comfort zone currently lies, take it up a notch. This is endurance training for your palate.

Beyond the antioxidant and health-giving benefits of more spices and fresh ingredients like tomatoes and jalapeños, you'll become more used to a broader spectrum of stimulation, and less exciting and often, less nutritional, ways of eating will begin to pale in comparison.

RECIPES

BREAKFAST: MEXICAN CHOCOLATE SMOOTHIE

I love this mixture of chocolate with a flavor fiesta. The cinnamon helps you with fat metabolism, and chili powder starts a metabolic bonfire. Today's smoothie should include 1 scoop chocolate Vega One or other protein powder; 2 teaspoons dark cocoa powder or a few squares of dark chocolate, 70 percent cacao or higher; a few shakes of cinnamon; and a pinch of chili powder or cayenne pepper.

SNACK: AVOCADO MASH

Get in more healthy fat and shake up your tastebuds between meals with this lightning-fast snack.

> half an avocado, pitted but not peeled
>
> sea salt
>
> hot sauce

With a fork, mash up the avocado inside its peel.
   Sprinkle with sea salt and a few drops of hot sauce.
   Eat it right from the peel with some lentil chips.

LUNCH: SPINACH-MANGO-CHILE SALAD

This take on Thai food includes mango to make the iron in spinach more bio-available and a tongue-tantalizing lime-chile sauce.

FOR THE SALAD

Drizzle of olive oil

1 cup protein of choice (beef works well here)

2 cups spinach

1/2 cup ripe mango chunks

1/4 red onion, sliced thin

2 teaspoons roasted pepitas (pumpkin seeds)

1 tablespoon chickpeas

sea salt and freshly ground black pepper to taste

FOR THE LIME-CHILE SAUCE

2 teaspoons olive oil

sprinkle of red pepper flakes

1 lime, juiced

1 teaspoon honey

In a medium-hot, olive-oiled pan, sauté your protein until browned. Mix the salad ingredients together in a bowl, and then plate.

Whisk together the vinegar and oil. Pour over salad, toss, and serve.

DINNER: JOLIE MAINE LOBSTER TACOS WITH DOS SALSAS
Serves 2

I chained myself to the bar until Davida, co-owner of Jolie restaurant, agreed to share this delectable recipe. Davida says you can make these with regular whitefish like tilapia, too, or anything else that catches your fancy. Steak, strips of portobello . . . you know the drill.

6 ounces Maine lobster meat (two tails)

FOR THE SALSA

1 tablespoon olive or canola oil

half a habañero, diced with seeds (These are uber-spicy peppers. You may want to wear gloves for this. Don't rub your eyes, just sayin'. Substitute jalapeño for less heat.)

2 tomatillos (green tomatoes), diced

1 tablespoon diced shallots

pinch fresh oregano

pinch fresh cilantro

1 teaspoon agave nectar

1 teaspoon low-sodium soy sauce or wheat-free tamari

1 teaspoon rice wine vinegar

10 strands saffron (optional, but beautiful)

canola oil

4 soft corn tortillas

clarified butter (recipe follows)

low-sodium soy sauce

2 ounces shredded red cabbage

Sadie's So-Easy Mango Salsa (recipe follows), optional

For the lobster

Bring 4 cups of water to a boil with a dash of sea salt. Add lobster tails. Boil for 5 minutes. Remove the tails from the water, and let cool for a few minutes. Remove the meat, and cut it into chunks about 1 inch thick. Set aside.

For the salsa

In a skillet, heat the oil over high heat. Add the habañero pepper, and cook for 15 seconds. Remove pepper to a paper towel to drain. Reduce heat to low, and sauté the tomatillos and shallots in the same oil. Remove after 15 seconds. Place the tomatillos, habañero, oregano, cilantro, agave, soy sauce, and rice wine vinegar in a blender, and blend for 30 seconds. Stir in the saffron and set aside in a serving bowl.

Final assembly

Heat a skillet on medium heat for 2 minutes. Drizzle canola oil in the skillet, and place two tortillas facedown for 30 seconds to brown. Flip the tortillas to brown on the other side. Repeat for a second set of tortillas. Place two tortillas atop each other on a serving plate. Sauté the lobster tail pieces in clarified butter for 30 seconds with a dash of low-sodium soy sauce. Remove the lobster tail, and divide it between the tortillas. Top with salsa(s) and shredded cabbage. Smile and serve!

CLARIFIED BUTTER

In India, clarified butter is called ghee and is considered extremely nourishing for your body and spirit. Use organic butter, it's butter . . . I mean, better for you.

> 2 sticks of salted butter

Melt the butter in a saucepan slowly until it boils. Let it sit for about 1 minute, and then skim off the foam that rises to the top. Slowly pour the butter out of the pan into a separate pan, leaving behind the milk fats that have settled on the bottom of the pan. You can strain the ghee again through a superfine strainer or two layers of muslin cloth if you want it really clear.

SADIE'S SO-EASY MANGO SALSA

Here's my quick mango salsa recipe to complement the regular salsa.

½ cup fresh or frozen mango chunks	¼ jalapeño, seeds removed (optional)
	half a lime, juiced
¼ red onion	

Put all the ingredients in a blender, and blend on Low until chunky and salsa-licious. Place in a separate serving bowl from the other salsa and serve.

BEVERAGE: FROZEN CUCUMBER-JALAPEÑO MARGARITA

This spicy-sweet delight is the perfect complement to your dinner. Sip with a clean, clear body—and conscience. Olé!

1 ounce tequila

1 ounce triple sec

juice of 2 limes

¼ cucumber, peeled

1 teaspoon agave nectar

quarter or half a jalapeño pepper, seeded and diced (keep the seeds in for more heat)

1 cup ice

Blend all ingredients together until icy smooth.

Serve with a sea-salt or raw-sugar rim, and garnish with a slice of lime and a sliver of jalapeño.

ACTION: THE SWITZERLAND TECHNIQUE

The Swiss have a reputation for remaining neutral in the face of world issues. I don't know if that's true, but if I had that much chocolate to protect, I'd stay out of it, too.

Sometimes we approach the center through the mind. Today we begin the journey with body and breath, and as you let go of resistance to reality, insights about how to bust a move from here should arise more effortlessly.

⁘ Come to sit in a comfortable position.

⁘ Place both palms on your lower belly.

⁘ Lengthen your spine inside your body, subtly activating the muscles very close to it, so it effortlessly waves upward as if it's seaweed climbing up from the ocean floor.

⁘ As you begin to relax everything around the spine, maintain its upward movement so that you gain deep core strength even as you
  • Breathe in to soften and expand the chest and then the belly.
  • Breathe out, moving the lower belly in and up to help press the breath out and massage the whole lower-belly area.

⁘ Pause and let yourself float in the silent spaces between each breath. Sit calmly, on pause, until your body naturally tells you to take the next breath. Spend 1 to 2 minutes on this step.

⁘ Once you feel more relaxed, either open your eyes and do the following exercise with your journal, or do it as a seated meditation:

- Bring your awareness to the experience you had that caused your suffering.
- View your situation from a more neutral place. Then
    - **Embrace what is actually happening.** Describe it as if you are a reporter taking notes for a story. Just the facts, ma'am. Notice when you blur the lines of neutrality with reactivity. Anytime you slide back into your fear-based story—aka "Everyone hates me now!!"—return to the breathing until you can come back to observer mode: "Someone is gossiping about me at work, and I just found out about it, so I'm feeling afraid that everyone hates me."
    - **Reflect from your Switzerland place.** Consider how it would best serve your Core Missions and maintain your personal integrity to proceed. Some options might be, in order of core-strength effectiveness,
        - I'm going to have a total panic attack and flip out for hours at myself and my loved ones.
        - I'm gonna march in there on Monday and tell everyone what she does on her breaks, Miss Lunchtime Martini!
        - I'm going to speak to my coworker briefly and let her know I know about the gossip. I'm going to tell her that if she has anything to say to me, I'd prefer that she speak to me directly. Then I'm going to go back to doing my own best work.

Now, open your eyes or close the journal, and go out there and take whatever action you feel best represents your integrity (even if it's inaction) from your new place of surrendered strength.

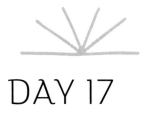

DAY 17

THEME: Stay Home

Today I have decided to focus more closely on the self-abandonment complex. Because if you're going to feel abandoned, it's helpful to remember who's doing it. You, not them.

Yes, other people can leave you. And it may seem as if they have caused the anxiety that ensues, the oh-please-come-back-I'm-not-OK-without-your-appreciation sensation that makes sane and capable people drunk-dial their exes at 3 a.m., run into snowy streets in bare feet screaming obscenities, or sell off all their cheating mate's personal items for one penny at a ga-RAGE sale.

In fact, that feeling has nothing to do with another person. "Abandonment" is a signal you generate when you walk away from your core relationship for the sake of anything or anyone outside of you.

We do this all the time, in large and small ways—for example, when someone doesn't text you back and you allow yourself to believe it's because you're not good enough, or you lose sleep cycling through some scenario that may or may not be happening starring your lover and a buxom blonde at a bar.

Self-abandonment happens when you stress out about someone leaving you, but have you ever noticed that it's always a good thing in the end when you find that next, more aligned situation—and more strength inside of yourself?

Notice when you feel abandoned. Are you engaged in an active process of ignoring yourself? Are you demanding that someone else placate your ego in order for you to feel like you matter? I'm not saying that you should love yourself more and at the same time put up with somebody who doesn't return your calls or value you. You're no longer going to love down a level.

Today let's begin to trade up.

Those old partners who couldn't fully love themselves (and therefore you) will become unattractive and old, demeaning relationship patterns will cease to hook you—because you have loved yourself up already and don't need to continue the cycle.

When your partner says, "I love you," it will be lovely—but not something you need to have in order to feel complete. Loving another isn't the cake, and contrary to popular belief, it's not even the icing on the cake. Because, honey, you're already sweet and complete.

There aren't any rules that work, no games you can play, to ensure that an external lover will love you well enough—or stick around. But you will always be there for yourself, so start developing it into an ironclad bond.

Today is a call to love, for you to reclaim your natural right to be the first line of defense, not against getting your heart broken by another but against you breaking your own heart.

YOGA

What we do to ourselves, we do to everyone else. That's why you must autocorrect behaviors that drag your own heart through the mud. If you met up with your friends and complained about your partner who just told you how stupid you were this morning, they'd tell you to kick him (or her) to the curb. Well, what if that person is you? You don't want toxic relationships? Then don't dish it in.

In our yoga poses, one way we self-abandon our core in order to offer our heart is by losing spinal stability and jutting the ribs forward in any pose, compressing the lower back and shearing the mid-back (thoracic) spine. I call this going to Thoracic Park. Not a good idea.

During your poses, keep your front top pelvic crests, front lumbar spine, and, now, front ribs drawing in and up, even as you express your lower-back curve and chest upward. Maintain your head in a natural curve, and you'll soon find out why, in yoga and in the world, we stay out of Jurassic Park . . . and come home.

Begin with 3 to 5 rounds of your Core Warm-Up.

Bridge between poses or flows with a Vinyasa sequence whenever you wish.

CUPID'S BOW FLOW

As so many transformational guides teach, the best way to love others is to love yourself. After all, like my homeboy Buddha said, there is no one in all the universe as deserving of lovin' as you. Not that guy or gal over there. You. When you do this, everyone benefits from your new, improved, inner offerings.

SPHINX

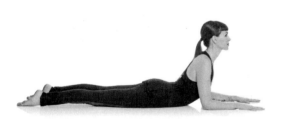

- Start in Downward-Facing Dog. Come forward into Plank, and lower to the floor on your belly.

- Place your forearms on the floor in front of you so that your shoulders stack over your elbows and your forearms are parallel.

- The palms of your hands are down, fingers wide.

- Point your toes and ground your feet down to charge the legs.

- Draw your front pelvis, rib cage, and spine into the front body and upward so that your tailbone and spine lengthen away from each other.

- Resist (don't move) your forearms back so that you get some traction in the lower back.

- Your shoulders and skull move back and up.

Breathe in Sphinx for 5 to 10 breaths. Press back to rest in Child's Pose.

CUPID'S BOW

- Come forward again to lie on your belly.

- Lower your forehead to the floor.

- Bend both knees, and reach for your outer ankles with your hands or a strap (a necktie or soft bathrobe belt around the feet will do).

- Press your feet back, and lift in and up along your front spine as your chest and shoulders stretch back and rise up.

- Move the skull back and up.

Take 3 to 5 breaths in Cupid's Bow. Move to Child's Pose. Repeat 2 to 3 times.

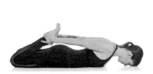 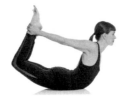 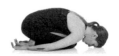

When done with Cupid's Bow, press back to Child's Pose for 5 breaths, and come into Downward-Facing Dog for Half-Moon Circle.

Half-Moon Circle

- Step your left foot forward, left fingertips forward and wide. Come into Half-Moon Pose.

- Take a few Half-Moon Circles: exhale the top arm back and down, bring knees together.

- Inhale, circle back up into the full Half-Moon Pose.

- Option: Next time you circle down, grab your right ankle with your right hand.

- Aim to open back up into Bound Half-Moon, this time with your right hand and foot creating a Bow-pose shape.

- Keep the top knee at hip level, and press your foot straight back behind you to increase this chest- and shoulder-opening backbend.

- At the same time, support with your Core Strength Muscle Meridian: move the front top pelvis, hips, spine, ribs, and face from front to back body and long through the crown—this will create a backbend, not a forward jut.

Take 3 to 5 breaths here, and then release the foot and stretch back into regular Half-Moon Pose.

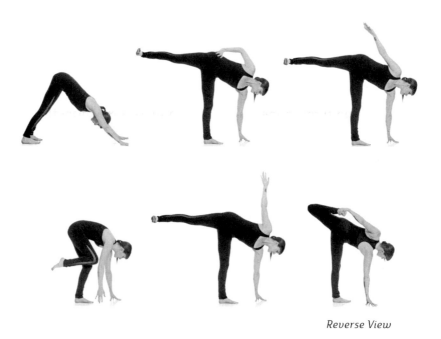

Reverse View

FAN-TASTIC FLOW

Fan Lunge

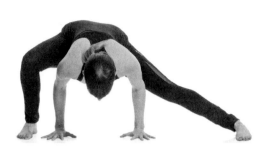

- ◦ Step your left leg back momentarily into a Warrior stance; then walk your hands to the center of your mat.

- ◦ You are now facing the left long edge of your mat with feet parallel.

- ◦ Bend both knees, and ground your palms or fingertips into the mat.

- ◦ Begin to straighten one leg and bend the other to stretch into the inner thighs.

  Repeat Fan Lunge a few times, spending a few breaths on each side.

Fan Pose

- ◦ Inhale, and press both feet down to straighten the legs to your edge.

- ◦ Wave up through the Core Strength Muscle Meridian: thighs, pelvis, belly, and down through the front spine and crown of the head.

- ◦ Exhale, and fold deeper.

  Take 10 breaths here.

Fan Twist

- ◦ Lift your torso up into a flat back. Stack your left hand on the floor or a block in line with your left shoulder.

- ◦ Spin your chest and left shoulder to the sky; then bend your elbow and place the back of your right hand on your back for

Half-Bound Fan Twist. Try to straighten your legs a little more here.

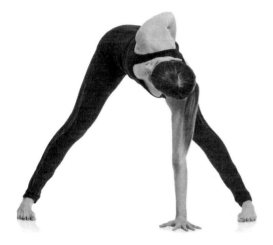

- Now flow it: Alternate inhale, twist up and straighten legs more, then exhale, roll back to face the floor with bent legs 3 to 5 more times. Keep the pelvic and spinal alignment long and natural; only straighten the legs to your healthy edge.

- Return to Half-Bound Fan, and twist your chest up to the sky one last time. Now unfurl the top arm to the sky. You should feel a lot more freedom in the shoulder.

Take 3 to 5 breaths here.
Return both hands to the floor at shoulder distance.

Fan Lunge here a few times, and repeat the Fan Twist on the other side.

Clasped-Hands Fan Forward Bend

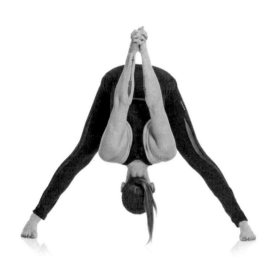

- Come to center in your Fan pose. Bend both legs.

- Bend elbows. Place back of your hands on your hips and internally rotate your arms, bringing elbows toward each other in front of you a little bit like you've got moves like Jagger. This "Jaggerasana" position roots your shoulders back more effectively.

- Still in Jaggerasana, slide your armpits and shoulders back.

- Now reach palms to face behind you. Clasp your hands, as you work to straighten your arms.

- Fold forward and stretch your hands farther away from your back to open shoulders and chest.

- Inhale, straighten your legs more, lift your belly up and over the legs and cascade length through your whole spine.

- Exhale and fold deeper.

Take 5 to 10 breaths.

Release your arms, bend your front knee, turn the foot forward, and return to Downward-Facing Dog. Repeat from Half-Moon Circle on the other side.

When you finish, end with your Core Cooldown.

Namaste! Good job today.

FOOD

Is your kitchen a place you inhabit, cooking up soul-food-filled, mindful meals? Or is it just the room you fly through like a bat out of hell on the way to work? Does your family see the dinner table as another workstation, a place to set the take-out containers, or have you created space to have regular family-bonding time there?

The ability to self-fuel and spark love and connection is directly related to how stubborn you are about making it a priority. What is more important than having a love-drenched, connective culinary experience with yourself or your loved ones? E-mail? *CSI*? Really?

Today, reclaim your kitchen as we focus on the belly-shui of home-cooked meals. You'll make dishes today that you could create for a life-affirming dinner party with your closest peeps, offer these meals as a gift to your family, or freeze them and free yourself from cooking on a few other days.

Today, get grounded in your own space, and prepare recipes that are made with reverence for health, from your heart.

RECIPES

BREAKFAST: BANANA-ORANGE-GINGER SMOOTHIE

This vitamin C and potassium-powered creation reminds me of a Creamsicle from my childhood. Note: You can always make more than you need, of this or any smoothie, and put the extra into freezer-safe cups to eat as a healthy sorbet dessert after any meal.

1 frozen banana, halved

juice of 1 orange

6 ounces coconut or almond milk

few drops vanilla extract

1 tablespoon flaxseed oil or half an avocado, pitted and scooped from the peel

handful frozen sliced peaches

1-inch piece of peeled fresh ginger, diced

water to reach your desired consistency

Blend all ingredients and enjoy!

SNACK: THE BEST GRANOLA BARS

Makes about 12 bars

Special thanks to my friend Chloe, who offered up her favorite recipe for the good of all man- and womankind. We salute you.

Making these takes some doing, but then you can store them in the fridge for a week or the freezer for longer and have them on-the-go whenever you want. Kids and adults alike love these protein-rich and fiber-filled bars that taste better than any granola bars I've had. They include chia seeds, which help sweep toxins from your digestive tract.

Crumble half a bar on your Greek yogurt and garnish with honey, or put it into a smoothie for some extra-credit chewy goodness.

2 teaspoons coconut oil for greasing the pan

2 tablespoons chia seeds

6 tablespoons warm water

1½ cups gluten-free rolled oats

1 cup shredded coconut flakes

½ cup vanilla protein powder (hemp if you can get it)

3 tablespoons poppy seeds (optional)

2 tablespoons ground flaxseeds

2 tablespoons sesame seeds (optional)

¾ cup chopped almonds, toasted

2 teaspoons cinnamon

¼ teaspoon nutmeg

½ teaspoon salt

3 ripe bananas

¼ cup coconut oil

2 teaspoons vanilla extract

3 tablespoons maple syrup

1 cup chopped dates (or any other dried fruit—I like dried cherries or apples)

Preheat the oven to 350°F. Grease a 9 x 13-inch pan with coconut oil. Set aside.

Combine chia seeds and warm water in a small bowl. Let sit for 5 minutes. Meanwhile in a large bowl, combine oats, coconut flakes, protein powder, all seeds, almonds, cinnamon, nutmeg, and salt.

In a separate bowl, mash the bananas with a fork until smooth. Add the coconut oil, vanilla, and maple syrup. Add the wet ingredients to the dry ingredients. Add the chia/water mixture and chopped dates. Mix thoroughly.

Spread in the greased pan. Bake for 20 to 25 minutes or until edges are golden brown. Let cool completely before cutting into bars.

LUNCH: ROASTED-ROOT-VEGGIES AND QUINOA SALAD
Serves 2 to 4

I had the most delicious roasted-vegetable dish of my life at my literary agent's house. I think she might have a second career here. Root veggies are known in ayurveda to promote a gravity of being, a precursor to love. So eat up—and ground down. Veggies that roast well include yellow onions, red bell peppers, zucchini, cauliflower, carrots, garlic, potatoes, and red cabbage.

1 tablespoon balsamic vinegar

1 tablespoon fresh or dried rosemary, finely chopped

2 tablespoons olive oil

2 cloves garlic, minced

1 generous cup each of five different, colorful veggies, cut into about 1-inch pieces

sea salt and pepper to taste

1 cup cooked quinoa

Preheat the oven to 375°F. Oil a 9 x 12-inch rimmed baking sheet.

In a small bowl, whisk together the vinegar, rosemary, olive oil, and garlic.

Place the veggies in a large bowl. Season with sea salt and pepper to taste. Pour the dressing over the vegetables, and toss thoroughly.

Spread the veggies evenly onto the baking sheet, and roast in the oven for about 20 minutes. Stir, and then cook for another 15 minutes. If you want them really crispy, you can always leave them in for another 5 minutes, but not much longer than that.

Mix the veggies with the cooked quinoa. Store any extra in the fridge and take with you to go for a couple of days, or freeze and reheat later.

DINNER: ROASTED TUSCAN LEMON CHICKEN WITH ROASTED POTATOES
Serves 4 to 6

This is a coveted recipe from one of the Don's friends in Italy. (Friend of a friend. Fuhgeddaboudit.) If you've got any leftovers, you can use them in pulled-chicken tacos or salad. Vegetarians, use the marinade with tofu or portobello mushrooms.

1 whole organic, free-range roaster chicken, about 3 pounds

¼ cup olive oil

zest and juice of 1 lemon

sea salt and cracked pepper to taste

1 medium yellow onion, quartered

1 sprig rosemary

4 sage leaves

4 cloves garlic

1 cup dry white wine (pinot grigio is a good bet), plus more (optional) for deglazing the pan. And drinking.

4 carrots, peeled and roughly chopped

2 stalks celery, cut into 2- to 3-inch pieces

1 medium yellow onion, peeled and cut into 8 wedges

1 tablespoon honey (or orange marmalade or raspberry jam)

sprigs of parsley, for garnish

Preheat the oven to 500°F. Rinse and pat dry the chicken inside and out.

Rub the chicken with olive oil inside and out. Mix the lemon zest, lemon juice, salt, and pepper in a small dish; then rub the chicken with the mixture inside and out.

Put the remains of the lemon inside the chicken, along with the quartered onion, rosemary, sage, and garlic.

Tie the legs and wings with oven string, and snip the tips of the wings off or cover with foil. Cover the drumstick ends with foil.

Place on a rack in a roasting dish in the center of the oven.

After 20 minutes, pour the wine into the corner of the roasting dish, and put in the carrots, celery, and onion wedges. Continue cooking for 40 minutes more. Check occasionally, and add water to the pan if it dries out, a cup at a time. When the chicken is cooked, remove from the oven, place on cutting board, and let stand, covered, for 15 minutes.

Place the roasted vegetables in a separate bowl. Pour some more wine or water into the roasting pan, and deglaze the pan on the stovetop for 10 minutes or so until reduced and thickened. It will be sour from the lemon, so add honey to soften it up.

Strain the sauce, and pour it over the vegetables. Carve the chicken into serving pieces. Put the vegetables in the center of a platter and place the chicken pieces over them. Garnish with sprigs of parsley and serve.

DESSERT: BAKED APPLE CRISP

Serves 4 to 6

After your dinner is done cooking, turn the oven down and throw these bad boys in. You'll be wowing your guests (or your own happy mouth) with this healthy alternative to apple pie. Make a few more if you want to have one left for lunch tomorrow.

4 apples, any kind you like	4 teaspoons agave nectar
6 tablespoons gluten-free rolled oats	generous sprinkling of cinnamon
	1 cup dairy-free ice cream (optional)

Preheat the oven to 350°F.

Slice the apples in half, and remove the core and seeds. Place the halves cut side up in a buttered baking dish big enough to hold them in one layer. Combine the oats, agave, and cinnamon in a bowl. Mix together until it's all sticky. Cover each apple half with oat mixture. If desired, drizzle with a little more agave and sprinkle with more cinnamon. Bake for 20 to 25 minutes. Serve alone or with some dairy-free ice cream.

BEVERAGE: SPICY LIMONCELLO LOVE

This is a healthy, sassy homage to the classic Italian liqueur, without all the sugar, calories, or alcohol. *Salute!* (Add 1 ounce of vodka for an adult beverage.)

1 teaspoon agave nectar for rim	juice of half a lemon (optional)
sprinkle of raw sugar	1/2 cup ice
dash of cayenne pepper	6 ounces sparkling water
half a lemon, cut into thin slices	1 teaspoon agave nectar to taste for drink

Squeeze some agave nectar onto your finger, and coat the rim of a tall glass. Then turn the rim lightly over onto a plate sprinkled with raw sugar and cayenne.

Muddle the lemon slices in a bowl with the back of a spoon. Add to the glass.

Squeeze the juice from the other half of the lemon in there if you love the pucker. Add ice and sparkling water.

Add agave for more sweetness if desired, though I like it plain and supertart.

ACTION: HOME-SHUI DAY

Is your home a place that heals and inspires you, or is it a frontrunner for an episode of *Hoarders* that drives you crazy and stresses you out whenever you're there?

The art of intentional clearing, cleaning, and placement of objects is called feng shui (pronounced fung-shway). Practitioners believe that the way you live—mindlessly or mindfully—has a direct impact on your health, wealth, career, family, and more. I can only tell you that when I did some very basic shui in my prosperity corner, I got an unexpected check in the mail for $100 the next day. Good enough for me!

Here are a few simple tips for ways to work some shui magic on your surroundings. Put some or all of them into action, starting today, and you may also charge up better energy flow in your most immediate environment.

Soji (soh-gee): This is the Japanese word for cleaning meditation. That's right—you can actually make mundane housework into a refreshing, centering Zen technique in which you think, "I'm clearing out all negativity from my life," as you wash the dishes or meditate on organizing your mind as well as your junk drawers.

Not many of us have hours to do one massive clean; however, twenty consistent minutes a day, in the morning if you can find the time, really adds up.

Money, Honey: I'm from Iowa, the "Field of Dreams," where we like to say, "If you build it . . . they will come." It so happens that this applies to money and all other forms of abundance, too. To catch more moneybees with honey, in the back left corner of any room, of your whole house, or even of your desk (what Black Hat feng shui theory calls the "money corner"), place some or all of the following:

- the colors of wealth: purple, gold, and green

- a jar of coins, which you add to often and also spend once in a while (after all, people with wealth don't have to hoard every little cent)

- photos or images that represent prosperity to you and things on which you would like to spend your money

- a lucky cat or Ganesh (the elephant guy) statue—both represent removal of obstacles and attraction of health and wealth

Bedroom Shway: The bedroom is a place for sleep, sex, and calm. The office should stay in the office and TV in the living room—not here in your sanctuary. Shift your bedroom into a soothing, sexy place with mellow colors, burning candles, art you love, fresh flowers, essential oils that make you sleepy, and the proper lighting, music, even a little bowl of dark chocolate that all conspire to get you, and keep you, in the mood for love and restfulness, instead of rest-less-ness.

I have a Himalayan rock salt lamp by my bed, which gives off a sleepy orange glow and healing negative ions, like the ocean! It's the best night-light ever. Look around the rest of your home during your sojis. Does it represent you, and if not, how can you clean it up, beautify it, and mirror your best self into your outer world?

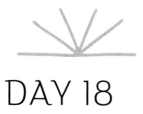

DAY 18

THEME: An Offer You Can't Refuse

I was teaching a class out on the road. Not *on* the road, specifically, but in a yoga studio on a cross-country tour. I was teaching the first steps to headstand, and everyone except one guy, who was way in the back row, was still on the ground in preparation. Maybe because he was new to the practice, he was already up, legs in the air, chin on the ground in this contorted bizarre *facestand* shape. I truly thought he might break his neck before I got back there to help him out of it.

As I hurdled over Downward-Facing Dogs toward him, I yelled out, like the Italian girl I am, "Hey, you! You better come down right now, or you're gonna wake up tomorrow to find a horse's head in your bed!" He somehow got himself out of the "pose" and sat bolt upright in his Easy Seat. (Luckily his head seemed to be resting at the right angle.)

The class laughed at my *Godfather* movie reference, but I was dead serious. (Not about the horse. I didn't even know where the guy lived, and plus, I'm so not a morning person.) My desire to get him away from possible injury and back into a healthy posture was strong. In the end, he was cool. He said he understood that I was trying to protect him. It probably helped that I was in Italian-centric New Jersey at the time.

When it comes to your own health, energy, and empowerment, I'm going to make you an offer you can't refuse (well, you can try, but after you do it my way, you're going to come right back to the Core Strength Family): Today, I want you to think veeeeery carefully about what you're going to say "yes" to from now on. Because your agreements and the actions you take from there can either heal you or destroy your vitality faster than you can say, "Leave the gun. Take the cannoli."

People in the business of transformation throw the word *empower* around a lot, but what does it really mean? Well, simply, it's a verb that is defined as "to give power to."

When you enter into any agreement with other people or with yourself, whether as simple as "Sure, I'll go get the kids from soccer" or as major as "Yes, I'll accept your job offer," you are really saying, "Here—I'm going to give power to you/to this right now." And I'll just say it straight: sometimes you leak your power, your life-fuel, away in ways that don't serve you, are destructive, or are just plain unconsciously arising.

Maybe you're saying "yes" to giving up your sacred sleep for obsessing about some stupid guy you won't even remember in two months. Or you could be agreeing to watch your neighbor's kids, when you hate doing it and it exhausts you, just so you won't have to feel uncomfortable during your next driveway conversation. There are no "noes," actually, only you saying yes to one thing or another. You're saying yes all the time. The question is: Is it serving you to deepen and evolve? Or not so much?

You could be fully participating in self-criticism or agreeing to smoke just so you won't gain ten pounds. So, are you saying "yes" to your healthy inner and outer yoga body or "yes" to remaining stuck?

Starting today, I would love you to make a pact with yourself to start honoring your "yeses." And make them fuel for your dreams, not water to dampen your flame.

When it comes to doing anything but offering on purpose, as uncomfortable as it might feel to decline to help, if you don't feel it's a healthy use of your time, energy, or skills, you can and will refuse.

In so doing, you are still saying yes: "Yes, I'm worthy of remaining balanced and full. Yes, I will commit to living in passion and love. And, finally, yes, I will make a contract with myself, one that stipulates that I can only choose to act on my own best behalf."

When you live according to this, your Big Yes, even if that "yes" looks like a "no" to someone or something, trust that you're making space for the person or thing meant to step into that role—and that the best possible outcome for everyone involved is assured.

YOGA

In yoga, "offering" into a pose more fully usually means you're going for the stretch, but there's a time when you've gone far enough and need to balance by containing yourself.

If you feel a stretch in or around your joints, you may be straining connective tissues, not stretching your muscles. Ligaments and tendons are your body's connectors, meant to anchor your bones, joints, and muscles in place: they move a little, but stretch them beyond their limits and they don't snap back—they just might snap.

Today as you express outward in your yoga postures, be aware of exactly where that stretch sensation is located. The safety zone is in the belly of your muscles. This is located around the middle of your bones, between the end joints of your muscles, for example, the center of your hamstrings, not the back of the knee or sitting-bone areas.

Today, you'll stay sensitive and exist both figuratively and literally in the core of your muscles. Bend your knees or come out of any stretch until you're back at center, and play your transformative edge gently instead of pushing too hard and careening over it like Thelma and Louise over a cliff.

Begin with 3 to 5 rounds of your Core Warm-Up.

Do 5 rounds of your Core Sun Salutations one after another to get really warm.

FLOW 1: TEMPLE DANCER

You'll start a lower body and root bonfire as you dance and release obstacles to your big "Yes": health, freedom, vitality, focus, love, and inner strength.

Side-Angle Dance

- ⁖ Begin standing in Mountain pose at the front of your mat.

- ⁖ Look down for balance, and step your left leg back into a Warrior stance.

- ⁖ Bend your front knee as your front toes turn forward and the back toes angle forward 45 degrees.

- ⁖ Spend the next 5 minutes rocking any moves here that you desire. I suggest some or all of the following:
  - Place your forearm on your thigh or take your hand to your ankle or the floor for Side Angle.
  - Release the arm up, circle it, half or full bind.
  - Triangle Pose.
  - Waterfall Warrior.
  - Fan Pose with arms clasped behind your back for a shoulder stretch.
  - Any other pose you feel your body is saying yes to right now. Trust yourself, get curious, and play.

Do Side-Angle Dance for 5 minutes on this side, and then continue to Twisted Lunge.

Twisted Lunge (shown here on the other side for easy viewing)

- Cartwheel your hands to frame your front foot. Spin your back heel up for Low Lunge.

- Place your left hand to the front left corner of your mat, stacked under your left shoulder.

- Root into the ball of the left foot, and power up your leg.

- Center your pelvis toward the floor so that the left hip doesn't sag.

- Wave long through your spine.

- Spin your chest to the right, and unroll your right arm to the sky.

- Pull the right hip back, and lengthen your left-side waist.

- Optional: try a Half- or Full-Bind around your front leg.

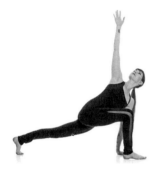 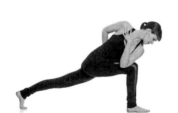 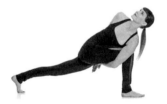

Take 5 breaths here; then begin Twisted Lunge Circle to Twisted Triangle.

TWISTED LUNGE CIRCLE TO TWISTED TRIANGLE

- Keep your feet and left arm as is.

- Begin to circle your right arm back down; exhale. Bend both knees.

- Inhale, and as you come up, straighten both of your legs more: ground your front big toe mound, pull the right hip crease back, and lengthen your spine.

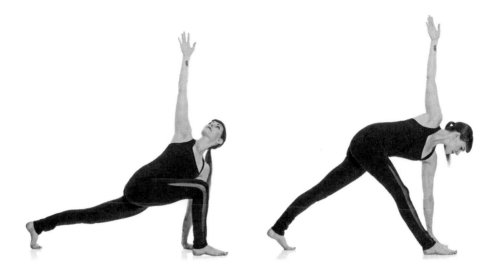

Alternate circling down and bending the knee with circling up and straightening the leg.

Circle 5 to 10 times; then move into Twisted Half-Moon Pose.

TWISTED HALF-MOON POSE

* Step your back foot forward, and reach your left fingertips forward until you can stand on your right leg with the left leg lifted parallel to the mat.

* Place a block under your left hand if needed.

* Keep the hips facing the floor evenly.

* Lift your belly and lengthen the spine.

* Begin to twist your chest and shoulders to the sky, and lift your right hand into the air.

* Look down to stretch the neck. Thread your top arm around the back for a Half-Bind.

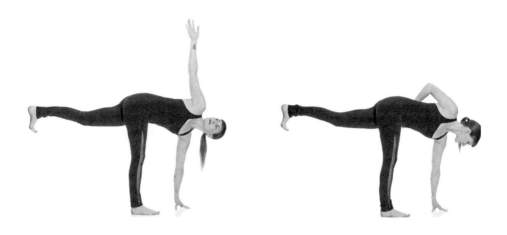

Take 5 breaths here. End in Standing Split.

Standing Split

- ⁖ Bring both hands to the floor, and center your hips again.

- ⁖ Inhale, and wave your spine long.

- ⁖ Exhale, and fold over your front, straighter leg.

- ⁖ Hang on behind your calf with the right hand if possible.

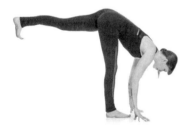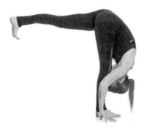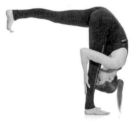

Take 5 breaths here.

Then continue into your Core Cooldown.

Hold Reclining Goddess, Pigeon Pose, and Seated Forward Fold as longer yin poses if you have time.

Namaste! Fantastic job today.

FOOD

When I first started switching my diet from processed to powerful, although the idea rocked, I felt a lot of resistance. After all, I don't like denying myself things I really want. That's not my idea of a life well lived. Then I realized that in saying "yes" to less quality, I was also saying "yes" to weight gain, poor health, and potential illness down the line.

We stop our progress with mismanaged yeses all the time, like buying pesticide-and-toxin-containing foods because organic food costs more. The way I see it, hospital stays and missed days of work, life, and love are far more expensive. So whenever instant gratification or a quick fix rears its head during your day, remember this: You're not saying "no" to anything. You can have anything you want.

You're not removing things. You're simply adding in actions that say "Hell Yes!" to health. Pretty soon, all your delicious Big Yeses will crowd out the smaller ones, and you'll be on the road to fit, fierce, and fabulous, faster. Today, with reverence, I offer you some recipes I adore from my closest family and friends.

As you prepare and enjoy these dishes, all of which have so much meaning for me, eat in gratitude for all the love, possibility, and supportive community in your life and for everything yet to come, and in so doing, say "yes," always "yes" to the delightful goodness that surrounds you.

RECIPES

BREAKFAST: GRANNY'S CINNAMON ROLL SMOOTHIE

I've loved cinnamon rolls ever since both Granny Nardini and Grandma Parrish made them for me as a child. These days, I create my own version in a smoothie that expands my energy, not my waistline.

1 frozen banana, halved

1 cup milk

1/2 to 1 teaspoon cinnamon

few drops vanilla extract

1/4 cup macadamia nuts

1/2 tablespoon flaxseed oil or half an avocado

1 teaspoon ground flaxseed

1 cup fresh spinach (optional; it boosts the nutrition, and you won't be able to taste it)

Blend all ingredients and enjoy. And while you're at it (the blender), . . . make the following snack now and freeze for later.

SNACK: FRO YOGI POPS

My mom used to make me yogurt Popsicles made of yogurt and Jell-O (loving attempts at health food, along with the less popular cottage cheese pancakes and spinach lasagna made with canned spinach), which we shall leave resting in peace back in the day. Let's give these rockin' pops a fresh update.

2 cups fresh or frozen fruit(s) of choice

2 cups Greek yogurt

2 tablespoons honey or 1 tablespoon agave nectar, or to taste

You can either throw the fruit, yogurt, and sweetener in the blender and puree it or, for a chewy surprise in each bite, stir the fruit and sweetener into the yogurt in a bowl. Pour or spoon the mixture into Popsicle molds. Freeze for 2 hours. Serve and lick!

Some of my favorite Pop-tails

strawberry and vanilla extract

raspberry-lime (juice of 1 lime)

mango-pineapple (dice 1 cup each fresh mango and pineapple)

cherry-blueberry

watermelon-lemon (dice 1 cup watermelon and add juice of 1 lemon)

LUNCH: MOM'S CHICKEN SALAD

Serves 2

My mom would rather be onstage singing French torch songs than cooking, so imagine my surprise one day when she whipped out this awesome chicken salad. Has she just been holding back on us all these years? Go, Mom!

2 to 3 cups rotisserie chicken, shredded

1 green or red apple, cored and chopped

1 scallion, sliced

1 cup seedless green or red grapes, halved

1/4 cup raisins

1 small stalk celery, sliced

2 dates, seeds removed and chopped

1/2 cup walnuts or almonds

1 tablespoon canola mayonnaise

sea salt and freshly cracked black pepper to taste

2 cups arugula or spinach leaves

pinch of brown sugar

Put all of the ingredients except the greens and brown sugar into a bowl. Toss with the mayonnaise, salt, and pepper. Arrange the arugula or spinach on a platter, and spoon the salad over the greens. Garnish with a sprinkle of brown sugar before serving.

DINNER: PASTA WITH LAUREL'S YELLOW OR RED SAUCE

Serves 4

Yeah, if you're busy, you could throw a jar of organic tomato sauce onto some pasta and be done with it. But there is nothing quite like making your own sauce and witchy-love-brewing it up for yourself and your family. My friend Laurel lives in rural Pennsylvania and gets her produce from the local farms. This recipe fuses Laurel's farm-to-table version with my more classic sauce from the Italian Nardini family.

If you don't have fresh tomatoes that you deem worthy of a sauce, you can save time and get 32 ounces of canned peeled whole tomatoes. Crush them with your hands right into the pot. Try a nonwheat quinoa or rice pasta with this dish.

12 large yellow or red tomatoes, as ripe as you can get them

¼ cup olive oil

3 to 4 cloves garlic, sliced

1 yellow onion, roughly chopped

1 medium carrot, grated

2 cups mixed veggies, chopped (celery, mushrooms, zucchini)

½ teaspoon salt or to taste

pinch of red pepper flakes (if you like it spicy)

2- to 3-second pour of red wine

2 teaspoons fresh or dried basil, rosemary, oregano or to taste

1 cup fresh spinach

1 to 4 servings of cooked pasta, depending who you're cooking for

½ cup grated Parmesan cheese

cracked pepper

Fresh basil leaves for garnish

Peel the tomatoes: To do this, poke each one a few times with a fork. (If you've got any aggression to let out, now's the time.) Bring a pot of water to a boil. Put the tomatoes in for under one minute. Remove from the pot and rinse in a bowl under cold water; the skin should come right off. If not, toss the stubborn ones back in the boiling water for another 10 seconds until the skin loosens up.

Cut the skinned tomatoes in half. Squeeze out the seeds over a strainer into a bowl to catch the juice.

Heat a pan on medium. Add the olive oil. Add the garlic, onion, carrot, celery, mushrooms, zucchini, and sauté for 3 to 5 minutes. Set aside.

Mash by hand or chop the tomatoes, and toss them into the now empty pot. Add the juice, too.

Wine 'n' Dine

Any good, full-bodied red is going to be awesome with your sauce, but my DNA compels me to go Italian with this dish.

Add the sautéed veggies, wine, and herbs. Then lower the flame and let simmer, stirring occasionally, for 30 to 45 minutes. Toss in the spinach in the last 5 minutes.

Serve over pasta. Garnish with Parmesan cheese, cracked pepper, and fresh basil leaves.

BEVERAGE: CHERRY GREEN TEA COOLER

This is a refreshing and enlivening alternative to coffee, and a way to get the antioxidant benefits of green tea in a new tasty brew. I suggest Republic of Tea Pomegranate Cherry Green Tea, but you can make a tea cooler with any tea you like and get creative with it.

1 green tea bag, plain or flavored

1 cup hot water

½ cup frozen cherries

splash of pomegranate or cherry pomegranate juice

ice

Brew the tea for 3 minutes; then pour into a freezer-safe container. Place the container in the freezer for 10 minutes to quickly cool.

In a tall glass, add a mash of frozen cherries and a splash of pomegranate juice. Add ice and the cooled tea. Garnish with a few whole frozen cherries. Enjoy your juicy energy drink!

ACTION: OFFERING ON PURPOSE

In a pleasant twist of financial fate, I'm considering making an offer of my own—on my first home. The question is: Where? I do love me some Manhattan, the only place that has earned the right to be called simply "the City," but then again, I'm partial to the clean, spacious country, too.

My decision remains to be seen. But let my story illuminate the big and small offers you are faced with all the time. The following is a technique I use often when I find myself in a conundrum between two or more choices.

The real question isn't what to do as much as *how you want to feel*.

What kind of inner experience do you want to have during your precious days—expansive or contractive, restrictive or free, core strong or depleted? Once you clearly see what *feeling* or *being state*, each potential choice leads you into, then you can direct yourself to reallocate your resources—financially, physically, and mentally in ways that get you the most bang for your being buck.

Consider using the following road map to navigate toward your own soul-smart decisions.

This, Not That

You want to make sure your agreements line up with the This side.

THIS...
It lights up my heart.
I want to do this.

...NOT THAT
It makes my chest feel anxious and tight.
I "should" do this.

| It's a win-win. | It's a win-lose (either for me or for the other person). |
| This fits my goals of health/happiness. | This keeps me stuck or moving backward. |

There may be other being-state deal-breakers that you want to add to your lists. Go ahead. Once it's complete, go sit somewhere that makes you feel comfortable. Bring your journal, and ask the questions about a small or large decision you've been pondering. If there's even one Not That that applies to your choice, it might be a deal-breaker. More than that is a dead giveaway.

Think not just about the decision in front of you but about other paths you can see that would not only be OK, but freakin' fantastic for you: the "Biggest Yes" of all. Write down what vision arises. Do you need to wait to choose until you get closer to that? Give yourself permission to be honest now without commitment to action, and you'll be much more likely to explore the best solution for you.

Once you can see what the choice is, don't talk yourself out of it just because you see (or are creating) challenges. Things have a way of working out when you're invested in doing what you were born to do.

Now create an Action Plan—and step by step, live your way into the new reality. You'd be surprised that, as Joseph Campbell said, if you begin to follow your bliss, doors will open where before there were only walls.

Trust this, and go forward. Ciao!

DAY 19

THEME: Joie de Vivre

joie de vi·vre \zhwa duh vee-vruhh\ n French: a delight in being alive; keen, carefree enjoyment of living

There is a very cool woman in my neighborhood. We'll call her Davida, because that's her name. As you might remember, she co-owns one of my favorite restaurants, Jolie, which means "beautiful." And she is. She wears unapologetically bright colors and awesome wrappy head scarves I could never pull off, and is basically a fierce muse who was born to inspire.

Davida is so full of life that every time I see her, I light on fire by default. When I pass her in the bistro, I always ask how she's doing, and without fail, even on the busiest day, she beams a high-wattage smile and says, "This is the best day *ever.*"

Davida chooses to focus on being a force of inspiration and positivity more often than she allows life to take her down. Much more. In fact, her new business venture is called If You Love It, Do It. That's also the tagline on every e-mail she sends. What kind of tagline would be on your e-mail to describe the world you're living in right now? If You Don't Really Love It—Still Do It Anyway?

When it comes to living, we're all (hopefully) alive, but what percentage of your day is spent immersed in *delight*? More than 80 percent? Didn't think so.

Let's improve that ratio. It is always my pleasure to do my best to guide you toward a state of joie de vivre whenever possible. And guess what? It's always possible.

Even if you're in the depths of grief, you can stay grateful that you have someone to miss and celebrate them instead of only grieving. My friend whose beloved husband died of cancer danced the night away with all her friends the night of the funeral. It was one great party.

Who says you can't laugh while you cry, can't splash like a child in a river of tears? To recognize your inner Alchemist, and transmute any and all experience into gold, you must remember to celebrate the wisdom and beautiful design of life, the sweet ebb and flow of it, and rock tears of joy as well as sadness. You do it *because* of what's happening, in honor of your experience, not as a way to avoid it. Here's what Davida said to me last time I expressed an urge to claim more of my own truth: "Yes!!! Do it, sister! *You have to be you!*" And so, dear reader, do you.

YOGA

Today, I invite you to practice more joie de vivre in your poses. You've trained your body to move from the ground up through the deep core muscle line. You can hold your focus more skillfully on the Belly Bonfire Breath to make sure you're invigorating that core heat. But can you do the hardest thing of all—give yourself permission to play with as much abandon as you did when you were a child? For this practice, I want you to *feel* more than you *think*.

We create these poses or structures not to dam our inner river but so that we can channel life force to ourselves and through ourselves without leaking it. So use your container in the way it's meant—for filling, and even overflowing, with a deep intention: to relax into your right to do the happy dance whenever you choose.

Dog Twist to Side Plank

You will warm up your arms and side core muscles as you balance, in order to create freedom all around your chest and heart center. Take your time in each move, breathing mindfully into the release, but have fun, too!

:• Begin in Downward-Facing Dog. Bend your knees.

:• Lift your heels, and twist the knees to the right for Twisted Dog.

:• Press strongly through your right hand, and breathe to stretch along your right rib cage and side waist.

:• Keep the knees turned to the right, and draw your lower belly in and up as you straighten your legs to come into Side Plank with one foot in front of the other on the floor.

:• Beginners: Bend your top leg, and plant that foot on the floor in front of you halfway up your mat.

:• Press your left hand and feet down firmly, and lift the hips away from the mat.

:• Lift your right arm to the sky if possible.

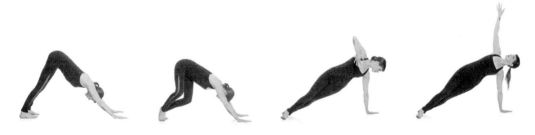

Begin to flow Dog Twists to Side Plank on each side 3 to 5 times.

On your last Side Plank on your right hand and leg, try Flying Triangle.

Flying Triangle

- Stretch your bottom (left) leg out to the right completely, and attempt to keep the foot and leg lifted off the floor for 1 to 3 breaths. Really squeeze and invigorate that inner-thigh party!

- Now, gently lower your outer left foot down on the floor, bring your right foot flat on the mat, and begin to press both feet down, lift your hips, and, if possible, reach your right arm up and balance on your left hand.

- Open your chest and top arm more, and fly high!

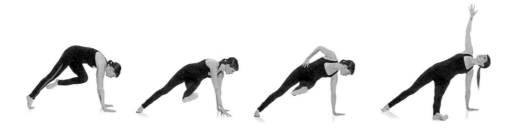

Hold Flying Triangle for 1 to 5 breaths; then return to Downward-Facing Dog, and repeat Dog Twist to Side Plank to Flying Triangle on the left.

Rest in Child's Pose and stretch your arms out in front of you for a few breaths whenever needed.

After your last Flying Triangle:

- Return to Down Dog with right leg lifted up into the air.

- Come to Core Plank, right knee into chest.

- Step your right foot into a Low Lunge.

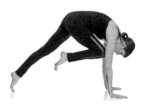
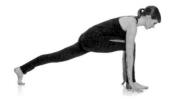

Flying Pigeon

- Step your back foot forward so feet come together at the front of your mat.

- Bend your knees, and roll up into Chair Pose. As you do, lift your left knee into your chest.

- Cross your ankle over the right knee, and bring your palms together at your chest for Ankle-to-Knee Chair.

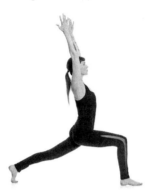 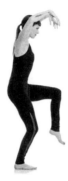 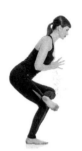

- Begin to reach your hands down to your shin, blocks, or the floor as you straighten your standing leg more toward an Ankle-to-Knee Forward Fold. Or, since today's a party, try this Super Adventure pose, Flying Pigeon:

- Maintain your ankle-to-knee position.

- Bend your standing leg, and plant your hands on the floor in front of you.

- Bend the elbows as if in Chaturanga.

- Try to hook your left toes around your right upper arm (have fun!).

- Press the shin into the upper arms while at the same time pressing the upper arms into the shins.

- Lean your hips and chest forward until your elbows stack over the wrists, and try balancing your back foot off of the floor.

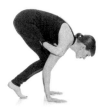

☀ If you're in it to win it, you could lift your left toes off the floor and then straighten the leg behind you so that you're hovering a Pigeon shape on your arms. Chip away at this—you'll get there!

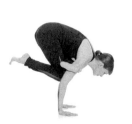

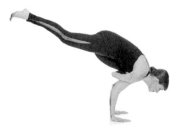

Come into a Forward Fold for a few breaths, and notice the difference you've made in your left hip and leg. Return to Downward-Facing Dog, and repeat the sequence from Dog Twist on your other side.

Then continue into your Core Cooldown.

Namaste! Très jolie job today.

FOOD

Speaking of joie de vivre, nothing puts a spring in your step quite like eating life-giveth (not taketh-away) foods that your body loves.

Today's recipes are all based around foods that amp your aliveness and literally illuminate you from the inside out. They work on many healing levels, but one that you'll notice, besides feeling invigorated and shiny, is that your skin will look fantastic.

Eat with gusto, and as you prepare and eat your meals, admire these simple ingredients. After all, they're giving their life force to enhance yours. Tell them how much you appreciate this, and eat in reverence for the ultimate offering of all things nourishing.

RECIPES

Begin your day with a hot green tea with half a lemon squeezed in it. It's a turbo-cleanse that will also clarify your skin.

BREAKFAST: FLAX-TASTIC HUEVOS RANCHEROS

Quick to prepare, these eggs give you a little kick in the asana to get you up and going in the a.m. Plus, the lycopene from the salsa has anti-aging benefits: it protects against UV rays and free radicals. The flaxseeds contain wrinkle-fighting omega fats, too.

drizzle of olive oil	1 teaspoon ground flaxseeds
2 tablespoons organic salsa	2 tablespoons refried beans
pinch of sugar (optional)	1 to 2 soft corn tortillas
2 eggs	few drops hot sauce

BONUS: If you're not going anywhere, or you're pre-shower, reserve a little of the egg whites and put on your face as you cook. You'll look strange for 20 minutes, but your instantly softer skin will be worth it!

In a medium-hot pan heat the olive oil; then add the salsa to warm. If you want it less acidic, add a pinch of sugar. Transfer the salsa to a bowl. Add a little more oil, and scramble the eggs by stirring constantly.

While the eggs are cooking, add the flaxseeds. Dollop the refried beans in a free area of the pan to warm. Remove the eggs and beans from the heat.

Heat another pan without oil on medium heat. Add the tortillas, one at a time if necessary, and warm for 1 to 2 minutes, flipping twice.

On a plate, layer a tortilla with refried beans, egg, and then salsa on top. Add a few drops of hot sauce to taste, and enjoy.

LUNCH: MISO-EDAMAME, BROWN RICE, AND KALE SOUP

The miso contains so many living nutrients already, but add the forty-five known flavonoids in kale and you've got an anti-aging, anti-inflammatory booster shot. Edamame adds protein, and half a cup has over half your daily folate, a B vita-min needed to repair your DNA! Now that's one power lunch.

2 tablespoons cooked brown rice

drizzle of olive oil

1 clove garlic, minced

1 cup mixed chopped kale leaves
   and edamame

2 cups water or to taste

1 tablespoon miso paste or to taste

Cook your rice, or use leftovers. Heat the oil in a pot over medium heat. Sauté the garlic, kale, and edamame until the kale is tender. Add the water, and bring to a boil; then lower the heat.

Place the miso in a small heatproof bowl, and add a couple of tablespoons of the hot liquid from the pot to make a smooth, thin paste.

Turn the heat off under the soup, and stir in the miso mixture until it is completely incorporated. Add the rice last.

Pour the soup into a serving bowl, and enjoy!

SNACK: SWEET POTATO FRIES AND CREAMY HUMMUS DIP PLATE

Both the sweet potatoes and the lemon in this dip are high in vitamin C, which boosts collagen. Olive oil's oleic acid softens the skin, and the vitamin E improves elasticity. And the zinc in the chickpeas helps repair your cells.

FOR THE FRIES

1 cup frozen organic sweet potato
   fries (can be found at most
   health food stores)

sea salt (optional)

freshly ground pepper (optional)

sprinkle of grated Parmesan
   (optional)

red pepper flakes (optional)

FOR THE HUMMUS

1 can organic chickpeas, rinsed and
   drained

1 lemon: juice of half a lemon or lime, plus
   juice of the other half for drizzling

2 tablespoons olive oil

1/2 cup Greek yogurt

1 clove garlic

sprinkle of ground coriander

sea salt and pepper to taste

cayenne pepper to taste

paprika, for garnish

Bake the sweet potato fries according to the package directions.

Season as you like. I add sea salt, pepper, a sprinkle of parmesan, and red pepper flakes to mine.

Put all the hummus ingredients in a blender, and blend to desired consistency.

Put 2 tablespoons or so of hummus in a bowl, drizzle with lemon juice, and add a sprinkle of paprika. Serve the hummus with the fries. Store the extra hummus in an airtight container in the fridge. Keeps for 3 to 4 days.

DINNER: ZAMAS' FISH WITH ANCHO CHILE SAUCE

Serves 2

I had this dish seaside at Zamas in Mexico and just had to share; the marinade for the fish can also be used on chicken or mix some into a dish of beans, veggies, and rice. Fresh garlic contains allicin, which helps you absorb the iron from the spinach and supports your immune system. The folate in spinach is also a well-known cancer-fighter, so throw an extra handful in your dish tonight.

FOR THE SAUCE

2 tablespoons olive oil

4 red tomatoes, chopped

3 green tomatoes (tomatillos), chopped

1/2 white onion, chopped

1 tablespoon chopped garlic

5 ancho chiles (Note: Each dried chile may be substituted with 1/8 teaspoon cayenne; but use the real deal if you can get them)

salt and pepper to taste

FOR THE FISH

2 (4- to 6-ounce) fish fillets like tilapia, mahimahi, or halibut

a squeeze of lime juice plus more for plating

pinch of sea salt

2 cups cooked rice

2 cups fresh spinach

sprinkle of cayenne

Heat the olive oil in a pan over medium-high heat. Add all the sauce ingredients, and cook until soft. Let cool for about 5 minutes; then transfer to a blender, and blend until more uniform but not pureed. Transfer back to the pan, reduce the heat to low, and stir occasionally.

Cook your fish over medium heat in an olive-oiled pan. A squeeze of fresh lime juice and sea salt should be all you need for seasoning.

On each plate first put a layer of sauce, then brown rice, then spinach. Place the fish on top to wilt the greens. Squeeze fresh lime over the whole dish, sprinkle with cayenne, and serve.

BEVERAGE: CANTINA BLOODY MARIA

Serves 2

Tonight, let's toast to Davida's indomitable spirit, and yours. I think it's only fitting that we whip up the heart- and skin-healthy mocktail/cocktail that Davida herself loves. This refreshing body and skin tonic (more lycopene!) is ready in 5 minutes and is perfect either with or without alcohol.

BLOODY MARIA MIX

10 ounces fresh tomato juice

1 teaspoon shredded ginger

1 teaspoon chopped cilantro

1 teaspoon grated fresh
   horseradish

1/2 teaspoon Worcestershire sauce

1/2 teaspoon Valentina Hot Sauce
   (or your favorite hot sauce)

1/2 teaspoon black pepper

1 tablespoon lemon juice

1/2 teaspoon chopped jalapeño

1/4 teaspoon balsamic vinegar

1 to 2 ounces organic vodka (optional)

GARNISH

2 cornichons

2 small jalapeño peppers, whole

Pour everything but the vodka into a pitcher, and stir vigorously with a long wooden spoon for 3 minutes. Add ice to glasses, and add any vodka. Add Bloody Maria mixture to fill. Spear one jalapeño and one cornichon each onto a toothpick, and place across the top of each glass. Sip and smile!

ACTION: JOIE DE SPA

Are you waiting for someone to hand you a spa treatment gift certificate? Why wait? Today you'll start transforming your home into a personal oasis where you can pamper yourself—anytime you please.

Here are three simple ways you can beautify on your own, using items you already have or can easily find, to bring on the bliss each day.

Bath Cocktails

I almost wrote, "I'm not talking about taking your champagne into the bath," and then I realized, that would be amazing! But I do suggest you dive into the wide world of creatively kicking your bath time up a notch. 'Tis so easy: in a metal loose-tea infuser ball, a square of double-layer cheesecloth, or a mesh sachet bag, put a mix of dried herbs, tea, spices, essential oils, or anything else you want to put into your bath but not get all over you. Once I tried to sprinkle in some loose spices and ended up rising out of the tub looking like the Swamp Thing.

Here are some of my favorite items to add (use fresh herbs when possible): Herbes de Provence, lavender oil, sea salt, grated lemon rinds, rosemary, peppermint tea, peppermint essential oil, sage leaves, bath salt, orange peel, clove, cinnamon sticks, ylang-ylang oil, grapefruit peel, grated fresh ginger, green tea, basil. Make sure to test a bit of any new oil on your skin first to make sure it won't react.

Fridge Facials

Nature isn't just a great nutritionist, she's a pro facialist, too. Here are a few beauty treatments that you probably have in your kitchen right now. Pamper yourself to one or more. Again, skin test these first!

EGG WHITE–LEMON MASK

Softens, clarifies, and brightens skin.

2 egg whites

juice of half a lemon

Mix the egg whites and lemon juice in a bowl. Apply to your face in gentle circles, avoiding eyes and mouth. Wait till dry, about 15 to 20 minutes; then wash off with a clean washcloth and warm water.

HONEY–OLIVE OIL–SUGAR SCRUB

Hydrates and exfoliates skin.

2 tablespoons olive oil

2 tablespoons honey

2 tablespoons white or raw sugar

Mix the ingredients together in a bowl. Apply to face in gentle circles, avoiding the eyes and mouth. Wait 20 minutes. Gently wipe your face clean with a warm wet washcloth. If you have any scrub left over, use it on your body in the shower.

AVOCADO-CUCUMBER-YOGURT MASK
Cools and soothes breakouts, tightens and hydrates skin.

half an avocado

half a cucumber, peeled and halved

half cup plain Greek yogurt

Put all ingredients in a blender, and blend till smooth. Apply to face gently. Wait 30 minutes until it sets; then rinse off in the shower or with a warm wet washcloth.

Go to the Ball

Why wait for someone else to massage you when two tennis balls will do the trick? Name them Ricardo and François, and go to town.

- Lie down on the floor on your back.

- Place two tennis balls at the base of your neck, one on either side of your spine.

- Gently inch yourself up so that the balls move down your shoulders and back. In time, you'll be massaging your lower back, which feels amazing.

- Pause and breathe wherever you find pockets of tension before moving on.

- Try the balls other places: glutes, hamstrings, quads.

Make a Joy Menu

To gather more joie in your vivre: write down the top ten things that bring you joy. Brainstorm how you can get more of those in today, and every day. Keep the list by your computer, by your bedside, on your desk, or taped to your mirror, and rock them out often.

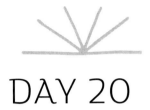

DAY 20

THEME: Open Your Whole Heart

After my close encounter with a hurricane in Mexico, I went back for another trip a few months later. And guess what happened? I got stung by a jellyfish. Right across my arm. It looked like *Fifty Shades of Grey* gone wrong: bright red stripes crisscrossing my upper arm and forearm, a spiderweb of burns that would last four months. Guess how I felt about this experience? Fantastic!

In my view, it wasn't bad. It's a *badge*—of honor. I had to be courageous and audacious enough to actually find myself in a beautiful ocean to be available for a jellyfish sting. Good for me! Maybe not so great for my arm.

So many people never dare to venture into the wide world—either to plumb their own ocean of Core Strength inside or to take a tour through love and mystery—because they're afraid it will go wrong and they'll get hurt.

Acting from the fear of pain doesn't save you from pain; it holds you back from the freedom to love, every time. You may have saved yourself from the potential of discomfort, but then you can't say you have truly lived—or loved, either. Regret hurts way worse than the temporary ouches of living out loud.

In case you haven't already noticed, when we defend ourselves from the idea of heartbreak because we're afraid to be hurt again, we don't avoid pain. In fact, suffering increases, because it expands into the empty spaces meant for intimacy and love.

In shying away from adventures of the heart, in refusing to stay openhearted, you make a statement to the universe that you are not willing, or worthy of trust or strength, which is far from the truth. You have the capacity to not only survive but thrive. Luckily, love is like LL Cool J: always poised for a comeback.

Instead of saying "I'll never trust again," be proud that you trusted, and loved with an open heart. Be discerning, and set calm, healthy boundaries—but do not make people currently in your life, or those you may encounter later, pay for the actions of others in the past.

This is a hallmark of a truly loving person, for it means that you believe your inner relationship is fulfilling enough, and that other people don't rock you to your core if they come or go. Then you're not afraid to love and love wisely, because you know that ultimately you can't really lose anything. No resistance, no regrets.

The second you decide to open more to love—the love you have within you and all around you—more love will appear. You can be in it, right now, beginning with the soul mate who's always been there for you and has never left. That's you, by the way, not someone you vibe with on an online dating site. Sure, let's not kid each other. Heartbreak bites. But do you know what bites harder? Not loving each moment that you can.

I have a huge crush on my own life and all those I draw near to me. Even if I decide that someone doesn't fit with me, or they decide it first, I can still move through that place of loss with integrity. (Plus, I get a lot more creative when I'm going through it. It's probably the Scorpio artist in me.)

What hurts far more than a broken heart is assuming your heart can be broken at all and closing off the natural state of affection and connection you have with the people you adore. If you truly love someone, love them as you let them go. Love them as you walk parallel paths holding hands. Love them if they falter, or if you do, and love them as you speak your truth. Most of all, remain unwavering in your true love for yourself, and you will revel in the experience of your whole heart.

Whoever comes and goes, there you stand. Because you loved yourself enough to fearlessly love another. You have fiercely, bravely, given yourself to love, in every moment. This is the hardest, most challenging yoga.

Because, in this life, the biggest victory isn't that everybody stays with you for a lifetime. It's that you have risked to love at all.

YOGA

We'll use your yoga poses to help you jump back on the Soul Train of Love today. Backbends are heart-openers, but it's so easy to overgive to them and lose your own core relationship. Everyone says "Open your heart! Love more!" but it's impossible to do that if you aren't fueling the belly flame that lights your heart from underneath—on or off the mat.

You'll leak your self-love and alignment whenever you jut the front pelvis, ribs, and/or the jaw too far forward, which sends the power of the pose straight out the front body and compresses the spine. When you channel your energy into backbends, keep it moving upward in one unbroken curve from root to crown.

Today, let's follow the central track that yogis call *shushumna*, the energetic banks and river of the spine and spinal cord. That's also where all three of your diaphragms—pelvic, breathing, vocal—stack in a line.

We'll maintain this healthy inner communication by focusing on aligning your spine: the healthy pelvic, rib, and neck curve that ensures you'll be giving your whole inner self some TLC, even as you reveal your whole heart fearlessly to the world.

Begin with 1 round of your Core Warm-Up and 3 to 5 rounds of the Core Sun Salutation to make sure you're really warm before you proceed.

FLOW 2: WHOLE HEART OPENING

To bring the body back to a new neutral from the backbends, let's open the entire chest and clear the throat, so you can enter all your relationships and express your truth with respect and love.

From Downward-Facing Dog, move into my Three-Pigeon Flow. You can skip the cooldown Pigeon today.

Waterfall Pigeon

- ❖ Come into Pigeon with your bent left knee forward and right leg back.

- ❖ Press your fingertips out to the sides and forward a little for support.

- ❖ Inhale, and roll your front body in and up to arch the chest with belly support.

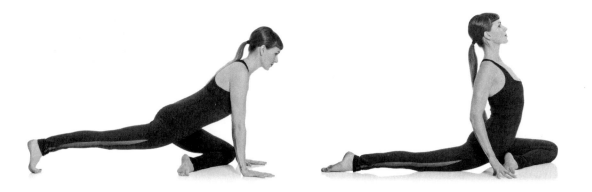

- ❖ Exhale, and lead with your chest as you pour the spine down and maybe touch your forehead to the floor or block.

Repeat Waterfall Pigeon 5 to 10 times, and on the last cascade down, move into Twisted Pigeon.

TWISTED PIGEON

❖ Place your right forearm on the floor or block, parallel to the front of the mat. Palm faces down.

❖ Inhale, and wave the spine long.

❖ Exhale, and spin the chest and shoulder upward.

❖ Look up or down.

❖ Bind your top arm around your back, or bend the back knee and take your right inner foot in the left hand. Bend the foot closer to the left sitting bone as you twist. Keep the hips centered.

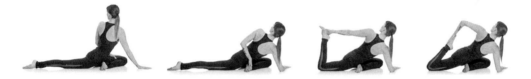

Hold Twisted Pigeon for 1 minute; then move into the last Pigeon to stretch the side of your heart and chest.

MOONWALK PIGEON

❖ Turn your chest to the floor, and begin to walk your hands or forearms over to the left, away from the front foot. Your spine is in a moon-shaped side bend, not a twist.

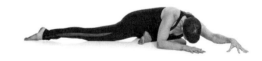

❖ Stretch your left arm out much longer, and breathe into your opening left side.

❖ If you want more of a leg stretch, scoot your front knee back an inch, and creep the right leg back a little, too.

Take 5 to 10 breaths in Moonwalk Pigeon.

Return to Downward-Facing Dog, repeat the three Pigeons on your other side. End with Stairway to Heaven.

Stairway to Heaven

This pose lets you restore with an open heart and aligned spine. The blocks help you keep the natural curve of your neck spine and save the orange juice for your mimosa.

- Take two yoga blocks, and near the back of your mat, place one block on a lower level and the next block one step higher. Cover with a blanket if you want extra padding.

- As you lie down on your back, the first block rests on or just under your shoulder blades.

- The higher block goes under your head.

- Let your arms rest at your sides.

- Place your legs in one of three positions:
  - straight out on the mat in front of you
  - knees bent, soles of feet on floor with feet nearly as wide as the mat and knees relaxing toward each other
  - feet together, knees wide in Goddess (place a blanket under each outer thigh here if you want a total restorative pose)

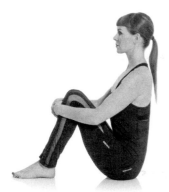

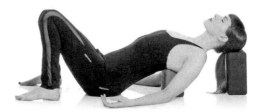

As your chest opens, and you rejuvenate your heart and core with the Belly Bonfire Breath, keep a light tone along the front of your lower-back spine to ensure the backbend stays out of compression and the energy is clear to move freely along your inner pathway.

Rest and receive in Stairway to Heaven for 1 to 3 minutes.

When you finish, end with your Core Cooldown.

Namaste! Such a heartfelt job today.

FOOD

When you look at a list of the communities in the world with the lowest incidences of heart disease and cancer, and the longest life spans, America isn't even above the fold. You'd think that with all our resources and medical knowledge, we'd be on top. At this writing, as far as life expectancy goes, we're number 30.

Heartbreakingly, many of those deaths are due to diseases that are diet-related and could be prevented, like diabetes, lung and heart disease, and some cancers. Let's bust this cycle and get with a menu of foods designed to both inspire your heart and heal it.

RECIPES

Nice Cubes In preparation for your final day's celebration tomorrow, sometime today, fill an ice cube tray halfway with water. Place an edible flower on top of each one, and freeze. If you don't have flowers, a single raspberry, basil leaf, or pretty little lemon rind will also do. When you wake up the next morning, fill the rest of tray to the top with water and refreeze to seal in the flowers.

BREAKFAST: CHOCOLATE-COVERED STRAWBERRY SMOOTHIE

This smoothie tastes decadent but is really just another healthy love letter from me to you, and from you to yourself! Lovely how that works. Make your smoothie and include the following:

2 teaspoons cocoa powder, or to taste (if not using chocolate protein powder)

1 square good dark chocolate

1 scoop Chocolate Vega One, protein powder, or chocolate milk

1 cup frozen strawberries

half an avocado or 1 tablespoon flaxseed oil

15 cups loving intentions

Blend and serve.

LUNCH: GREEK QUINOA SALAD

This breezy take on a classic Greek salad gives your heart even more TLC with the fresh ingredients, olives, and olive oil that one of the world's healthiest populations swears by.

1/2 cup cooked quinoa

1/4 cucumber, diced

1 cup salad greens (watercress is amazing)

1/4 cup fresh chopped tomatoes

1/8 red onion, diced

8 Kalamata olives

crumbled feta cheese

drizzle of olive oil

drizzle of red wine vinegar

sea salt and pepper to taste

few shakes dried oregano

In a large salad bowl, toss the first seven ingredients with olive oil and a hearty splash of red wine vinegar. Add the sea salt, pepper, and oregano to taste, and toss again.

DINNER: WHITE BEAN AND BRAISED KALE SOUP

Serves 2 to 4

This might look like soup. It's not soup. It's a reason to live. You can find the longer, soak-the-beans, make-Italian-grandmothers-proud version at www.21Day YogaBody.com, shown by The Don himself. But here's a quick, Sadie-fied version.

2 cans organic cannellini beans, rinsed and drained

4 cups chicken stock or vegetable broth

3 to 4 fresh sage leaves

2 cloves garlic, peeled

½ medium carrot, peeled

½ medium yellow onion

¼ cup fresh parsley leaves

½ stalk celery

2 tablespoons organic virgin olive oil

⅛ cup tomato paste

2 cups chopped kale

4 cups water

sea salt and pepper to taste

1 loaf Italian or gluten-free bread

sprinkle of Parmesan cheese

Place the beans in a medium-size pot, and cover with the stock. If the stock does not completely cover the beans, add some water until they are covered.

Put the beans over a low flame, and add the sage leaves and garlic. Simmer for 10 minutes, or until thoroughly warmed. Remove from heat.

Chop the carrot, onion, parsley, and celery roughly to fit into a food processor or blender, and then process for 30 seconds or until finely chopped but not mushy. Heat the olive oil in a 4-quart pot (the heavier the better for even heat distribution) over medium heat.

Pour the vegetables into the pot, and sauté over low to medium heat until the liquid evaporates.

Add the tomato paste, and mix well. Add the chopped kale leaves, and braise for 10 to 15 minutes. Add a ladle of the bean liquid, if necessary, to keep the vegetables from drying out.

Add the water, and bring to a boil; then turn the flame down to low, cover, and let simmer, stirring occasionally, for 20 minutes. Add more liquid as necessary.

Put half of the cooked beans in the food processor, and puree with just enough liquid to keep them moving smoothly. Using a rubber spatula, scoop the pureed beans into the soup pot.

Add the remaining beans and liquid to the soup, and simmer on a low flame for another 25 minutes. Add salt and pepper to taste.

As the soup cooks, grill slices of bread in a little olive oil and sea salt in a medium-hot pan. Set 2 to 3 slices in the bottom of each bowl. Ladle soup over the bread. Drizzle with your best olive oil, and garnish with Parmesan cheese.

You can make this filling dish in about an hour. It's great to take to work, so we'll make enough to freeze! Have it solo or with a sautéed protein of choice. If you're really pressed for time, throw everything but two cans of beans and kale in the blender (you might need to do this in batches). Blend roughly, toss in a pot with the beans and kale, and simmer for 10 to 20 minutes. I won't be able to face Don, but hey—you'll get to bed on time.

BEVERAGE: ROOIBOS TEA

Long renowned in Africa for its healing powers, this tea boasts high levels of antioxidants and flavonoids, like green tea, but it's naturally caffeine free. It's also thought to aid fat metabolism and vitamin C absorption. Your heart—and whole body—will love this. Drink hot or iced, with a squeeze of lemon.

ACTION STEP: CHOOSE YOUR ADVENTURE

One thing I've come to understand, after saying a wholehearted "Yes!" to enough adventure, is that it always, always leads you where you need to go. If you really want to do something, and it feels right in your body and spirit to see it through, you can and will find a way.

Forget about dreaming big. Dream massively. There's very little competition there, since so many people don't believe in their own possibilities, and they're busy thinking small. Make yours the most beautiful, expansive dream you can while you're here. Today choose your own adventure. Open your mind to it, keep an eye out for it, and then rock it like a hurricane when it shows up.

Your mission is simple: Today, do one thing—eat it, listen to it, or whatever—that you have never tried before. Do it as big as possible. You might . . .

- Jump out of a plane (What? You could! Just don't forget the parachute).

- Make the first move.

- Eat at a new restaurant.

- Veer into the park you always rush past on the way to work, sit for five minutes, and soak in nature.

- Grab your camera, and spend the day walking around and capturing all the cool little artistic details you may have missed while you were focusing on the bigger picture.

- E-mail your idol and ask for advice . . . or a job.

- Dress up twice as much as is necessary for any outing.

- Dance with abandon, but please, try something besides those same "running man" moves that were funky-fresh in high school; they have now expired.

Whatever you do, do it soon! Resistance may arise, but massive transformation is waiting on the other side.

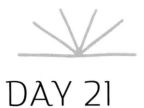

DAY 21

THEME: BE *HER*, NOW

I've always loved discovering a new restaurant, so right now, I'm in heaven. I'm dressed to the nines, having a cold glass of Gruner Velt-liner, one of my favorite whites, and contemplating spending more than my rent for a sirloin steak with blistered peppers and enoki mush-rooms.

I decide that having a roof over my head next month isn't all it's cracked up to be, order the gorgeous steak, send an Instagram photo of it to my peeps, tag it #foodporn, and then open my Moleskine and start writing these words. But as it happens, I'm interrupted, sweetly, by the bartender. She's looking at my pages and asks, "Are you a writer?"

"Why, yes," I reply. "I am."

Now, even if I didn't have a book deal, I can, and do, answer this same way on most given days. You know why? Because I'm writing.

And as you, beloved, are about to move from this program out into your world again, one of the most important talismans to carry for-ward with you in order to live the most charmed life possible every day is to know this: there is nothing as satisfying as being creative, simply for its own sake.

I'm equally happy writing in a local café or filming a free podcast for YouTube as I am if someone decides to make a TV show with me. I can say this honestly, because I've had it both ways. Don't get me wrong: I'm grateful for the opportunities that I have, but I don't need them in order to be immersing myself in storms of spirit and lighting bonfires of *muse*mallow-toasting, self-expressive *s'mores*.

Regardless of what comes of your efforts, or how much money you have, it is completely within your power to live as the artist you are, every day.

Too often, we wait—for someone to tell us we're good enough to sing, dance, paint that canvas, rock the casbah, whatever. And every day that you wait for an audience, or even someone to tell you that your work is worthwhile, is, in my opinion, a tragedy of Shakespearean proportions. Or at least a total creative buzzkill. A day not fully lived is one you'll never get back again.

When it comes to time, there are no do-overs. Starting today, throw out any care about what will happen to your creations, or who will like them, and just create. Refuse to use your days for things that don't rivet your attention, slow down time, or make you feel sizzlingly alive.

Find any and every way to be the artist, the lover, the adventurer, and spend your precious time on passion projects instead of worrying about what you cannot control—such as whether anyone will get it or appreciate you for your efforts.

The more I focus on the joy of my work, the more opportunities arrive, giving me the chance to turn them into something from which other people may benefit. Although I might have a goal in mind, and do things like pitch my ideas to network executives or reach out for outlets to publish my writing, this is all really extra credit. I'm already satisfied.

Then, next time you're engrossed in your own moment of mad musefulness, and if someone asks you if you're an artist, you, too, can smile and say, "Yes, I am."

YOGA

I reflected on what should be my last offering of this book to you. So here goes: All of yoga and life is a constant dance between opposites.

We work, we rest, we laugh, we cry, we become dazed and confused, we figure things out. We strive to evolve yet aim also to accept and honor ourselves just as we are. In the end, and the beginning, both of which you are experiencing today, no one can tell you what the right path is for you, not even me.

Ultimately, no one's trajectory moves along the same lines as yours. So, if others don't automatically understand or agree with your vision or choices, it doesn't mean it's wrong for you. It's just not right for them.

Today, let this free you even more to create your yoga practice in the way you feel is best to move into your unique dance of balance. Yogis call this ever-morphing spectrum *sthira-sukha* (stheer-a, sookha), or strength and ease, stability and mobility, support and freedom. Somewhere between the two, you'll find yourself.

For the last practice of this program—but I hope just another practice in your new fit, fierce, and fabulous lifestyle—I invite you to choose any of the 21 flows you love or to make it up as you go. Dance, sing, step off your mat, design new poses that work for your body. Basically, if you've been operating inside of a box, then go on and bust out of it, or at least go get a bigger box.

Spend 20 to 30 minutes or more in your practice today, as you cha-cha with this moment and swing into celebration of your Yoga Body adventure and all the inner strength and outer freedom you've revealed.

In honor of your off-the-hook artistic potential, I'll offer you two of my favorite moves—"canvas" poses onto which you can paint your personal masterpiece moment. Take them on, and then, as Madonna said, express yourself!

To celebrate your amazing 21-day achievement, bust a move with a 2- to 5-minute Dance Party!

Put on your favorite dance songs (I suggest Pandora.com's Dance Club station), or just move to your inner beat, and shake what your momma gave you for at least 2 minutes. No holding back, no looking around to see who's watching. Then come to sit and get mindfully wild with Wild-Angle Pose.

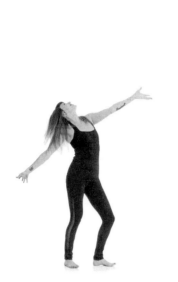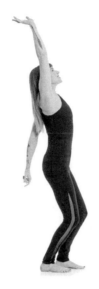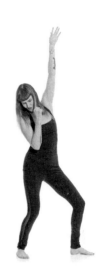

Wild-Angle Pose

⁛ Come to sit with legs wide, like a Fan Pose on the floor.

⁛ Flex your feet so that your toes face the sky.

⁛ Plant your fingers on the floor behind you.

⁛ Activate your legs so that the heels press down and your legs try to straighten. Remember, the pelvic and lumbar alignment is sacred. So, if your legs stay bent, so be it—just charge them up.

From this position, try one or more of the following variations, or make up one of your own.

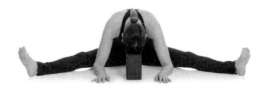

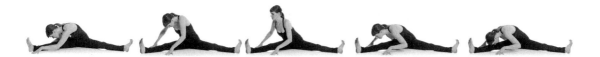

Spinal Wave Forward

- ❖ Inhale, root your seat, and wave the spine long.

- ❖ Exhale, and begin to hinge forward into the stretch.

Do the Spinal Wave 5 to 10 times slowly.

SPINAL WAVE SIDEWINDER

- ❖ Move like a sidewinder snake, letting the rib cage on one side lead you left and then the other right.

SIDE STRETCH

- ❖ Hook your right elbow inside the right knee.

- ❖ Side bend, reach your top arm for the straight leg's foot. As an option, lift your hand up to your head and rest your head in your right fingertips.

- ❖ Stretch your left arm over the ear more as you root your left hip down for a juicy low back and side spine releaser.

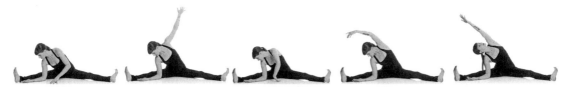

YANG FOLD FORWARD HOLD

- ❖ Fold forward over both legs, and then center. Hold for a few breaths.

- ❖ Hinge forward, keeping legs bent if needed.

- ❖ Maintain active muscles by pressing your legs into the mat.

YIN-IT-TO-WIN-IT HOLD

- ⁕ Stay in forward fold, but make it a yin-balancing pose.

- ⁕ Bolster under your chest and head with a stack of pillows.

- ⁕ Feel a light stretch in your muscles and joints.

- ⁕ Relax all of your muscles, and rest your cheek to one side or the other.

  Breathe here for 3 to 5 minutes. Then move into Belly Roll.

Belly Roll

This amazing pose is an uber-restoring, detoxing, and mellow sleep-promoting powerhouse that releases serotonin, otherwise known as your happy chemical. Over 90 percent of serotonin is produced in your digestive tract, not in your brain. So let's get in there and use your inner pharmacy to free up an actual sense of inner peace and satisfaction, and with it, restore your creative freedom.

- ⁕ Take a dish towel. Open it completely, and begin to squish and roll it into a little ball—about the size of a grapefruit or softball.

- ⁕ Lie down on your belly, and place the ball in the soft lower belly—midway between your navel and pubic bone.

- ⁕ The ball is inside the hip bones, so they don't rest on it but rather drape over and around it.

- ⁕ Place your cheek on your forearms or the floor, and rock slowly and gently from side to side to let the ball deepen into your belly.

- ⁕ Inhale into the ball more.

- ⁕ Exhale, relax, and allow the ball to go deeper.

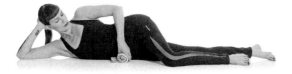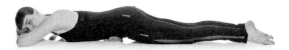

Be in the Belly Roll for 5 minutes, unless you get really nauseous. You could be pressing on an artery or have just eaten, and it's not a good combo.

You can try a smaller ball, and if that doesn't help, do this for less time until you can work up to 5 minutes.

Then continue with your Core Cooldown. Namaste!
And congratulations—you finished Day 21! Woohoo!!

I recommend doing the Belly Roll every other day and before bed anytime you need help getting to sleep and sleeping more deeply.

FOOD

Today is a throw-down, power-up celebration. Are you as worthy of artistically presenting a beautiful meal to yourself as to a guest you're trying to impress? With each creative action, on or off the table, are you representing the best you to the outside world? You don't do this for others as much as you do it just to align the most fully to who you were born to be. When it comes to becoming your own meal muse and making life look, and taste, just a little more gorgeous, let's testify—and beautify! Holla!

RECIPES

BREAKFAST: G-FORCE SMOOTHIE

This is an offering from Gabriella, my good friend and holistic health advocate. This smoothie, like her, is a creative force of nature, and is rich in potassium, antioxidants, anti-inflammatories, and omega-3 fats. It's guaranteed to propel you into your day like rocket fuel.

8 to 10 ounces coconut water

3/4 cup chopped kale

1 cup frozen dark cherries or berries

1 teaspoon organic coconut oil

1 to 2 tablespoons raw almond butter

1/8 teaspoon cinnamon

Blend and enjoy!

SNACK: KOKOPELLI KALE CHIPS

Gabriella also gives us this spicy snack, loaded with inflammation-fighting antioxidants and flavonoids plus vitamin K for bone strength. It is inspired by Kokopelli, a healer and god of music sacred to southwestern Native Americans. He is always shown in celebration, perfect for the one you're having today, in your life—and in your mouth!

1 bunch kale, rinsed and dried, stems and ribs removed

2 to 3 tablespoons extra-virgin olive oil

1 teaspoon Himalayan or sea salt

1 teaspoon chipotle powder

1 teaspoon crushed red pepper flakes

Line a baking sheet with parchment paper, and preheat the oven to 275°F. Chop or tear the kale leaves into 2-inch pieces. In a large bowl, toss the kale with olive oil, sea salt, chipotle powder, and red pepper flakes. Coat the leaves evenly, and spread them out onto the lined baking sheet.

Bake until crisp, turning as needed, about 15 to 20 minutes. Store in an airtight container on the counter. Crunch and munch, or crush and add as a delicious topping to soups or salads.

LUNCH: CARAMELIZED PEPPER-WALNUT PEAR SALAD

Let's celebrate this beautiful union of whole and tasty that no one can tear asunder. Treating the walnuts with an extra bit of care and using maple syrup instead of corn syrup or table sugar is a healthy shout-out in every bite.

Make a salad, and include a sliced half of a pear, a crumble of goat cheese or blue cheese, and dried cranberries. Garnish with a few of the pepper-walnuts, and serve!

2 cups walnuts

1/3 cup maple syrup

dash cayenne pepper (optional)

1/8 teaspoon sea salt

few shakes cracked black pepper

Preheat a dry skillet over medium-high heat. Add the walnuts, maple syrup, cayenne, salt, and pepper. Stir continually as it cooks, about 3 minutes. Transfer the walnuts to a waxed paper–lined or nonstick baking pan to cool. Once cooled, crumble the walnuts into a covered container; store extra in fridge. Keeps for a few days.

DINNER: BURGER NIGHT!!!

Serves 2

One of my favorite times in Brooklyn was when my bestie, Ava, and I would meet for organic beef burgers and wine at a local farm-to-table bistro. Here are my favorite burgers, with a side that replaces fatty fries for the better.

2 burger patties (try premade organic ground beef, lamb, buffalo, turkey, or ostrich patties, or rock one big portobello mushroom—the vegetarian burger!)

2 teaspoons Shake 'n' Serve Light Vinaigrette (page 18)

sea salt and pepper to taste

olive oil

2 eggs

squirt of Dijon or stone-ground mustard and organic ketchup

2 burger buns, gluten-free or whole grain

half an avocado, sliced

a few thin slices red onion

a few leaves of salad greens

Marinate the meat or mushroom in a bowl for 2 minutes on each side in the Shake 'n' Serve Light Vinaigrette. Add salt and pepper to taste.

Cook in a medium-hot, olive-oiled pan, flipping every 4 minutes until browned and cooked through. If using a portobello, flip every 2 minutes until browned on both sides.

Drizzle olive oil in another medium-hot pan, crack in 2 eggs, and cook without flipping until they reach your desired consistency from over easy to over hard.

Spread mustard and ketchup on both insides of a gluten-free (when possible) bun. Layer the bottom bun with the avocado slices, burger, red onion, lettuce, egg, and the top of the bun, and serve with Mange-Tout (recipe follows).

Wine 'n' Dine

Burgers are great with lots of things, but Ava and I enjoy this meal with an affordable, meaty Chilean Carménère.

MANGE-TOUT (MANDGE-TOOT, OR "EAT IT ALL," IN FRENCH)

Add my favorite side in place of fries if you want. It takes 4 minutes.

2 cups frozen or fresh sugar snap peas

1 tablespoon olive oil

1 to 2 cloves garlic

fresh ginger, peeled and finely grated

If necessary, snap the ends of the peas off with your fingernails.

Heat the olive oil in a medium-hot pan.

Sauté the garlic until light brown.

Toss in the peas, and stir occasionally for about 3 minutes.

During the last minute, sprinkle the grated ginger over the peas. A little goes a long way.

DESSERT: PEAR/BERRY CRISP

Serves 2

You can also crumble the topping for this recipe onto simple baked apples or pears, or use it as a crunchy complement for hot or cold cereal in the morning.

FOR THE CRISP TOPPING

1/3 cup gluten-free quick-cooking oats

1/3 cup organic raw sugar

1/4 teaspoon sea salt or to taste

1 teaspoon ground cinnamon

1/4 teaspoon nutmeg

1/2 cup chopped nuts (I prefer walnuts or pecans)

6 to 8 tablespoons unsalted butter, melted

FOR THE FILLING

3 cups peeled, cored, and sliced pears

1 cup blackberries

1/3 cup sugar or agave nectar

2 tablespoons cornstarch, tapioca, or arrowroot starch (I often leave this out and go au naturel)

1/2 cup gluten-free flour (I use quinoa flour; you can also grind some of your uncooked quinoa in a washed coffee grinder if you want to make it fresh)

Preheat the oven to 375°F. Grease a 2- to 2¹/2-quart baking dish or deep pie dish.

Make the crisp topping first. Blend all ingredients in a blender (pulse on Low) until crumbly but well mixed. Set aside in a bowl.

Combine the fruit, sugar or agave, thickener if you're using it, and flour in a bowl, and stir gently. Put the fruit mixture into the baking dish, and cover evenly with the crisp topping.

Bake for about 30 minutes or until the top is browned.

Serve solo or with an organic or dairy-free ice cream. Caramel, cinnamon, straight-up vanilla, or chocolate ice cream would all be wonderful with this dessert.

BEVERAGE

Take those flowery Nice Cubes you made yesterday out of the freezer, add them to a glass of sparkling wine or water in a flute glass, and toast to yourself and your journey through these past 21 days. This kind of courage is rare and wonderful, and you deserve every bit of recognition for your accomplishment.

CONGRATULATIONS on becoming a true Yoga Body Rock Star!

ACTION: BE WHAT YOU'RE BECOMING

A lot of people just deal with the reality that's right in front of them and work with that. It's understandable. You've got responsibilities, bills to pay, and a routine based on what you created up until now.

You can go retro all you want, yet if you want to move forward in any meaningful way, it's helpful to focus your attention on where you are, yes, but also where and who and what quality of life you want to be living in six months or a year or just in general. Is this somehow different from what's going on now? If so, begin to create space for the future to pour in, in the form of being that way, today.

Ava, my burger buddy, wanted an office space in NYC and found one in a cool office-share created for women. Yet she still envisioned having her own, personal, more private desk in the VIP offices a floor down. She asked the receptionist if there were any available desks. When the receptionist replied "No," Ava asked, "Can I go look at them anyway? I just like to put my vision out there, and you never know what will happen." The receptionist took her down, and Ava set her mind right then and there on having one of those desks someday. She even went out and bought a vase for "her" desk and planned out how she would arrange it when the time came. Well, the time came . . . twenty-four hours later! She got a call: someone was leaving suddenly, and did she want the desk—with a view even? Best desk in the place. On this day, I invite you to begin to look, ask, plan ahead, and start acting like the person you wish to become.

Create a void in the shape of your best life, and it will pour in to fill it. If you want prosperity, start giving what you can for free, as if you didn't need the money (I did this with my YouTube videos, and still do), or become more generous in spirit. Start treating the money in your wallet with care, and thank every dollar that comes to you.

If you want a relationship, then put out a glass of wine and a plate for this person when you fix one for yourself. Clear out a drawer for their future stuff. Make an extra house key. Envision them in your life. If there's a goal you want to meet, start acting on it now. Take any little or big steps that may potentially move you closer to it. Make a vision board, bring your coffee from home, and then put the $4 a day you would have spent on your latte into a "Dream Fund." There is always something you can do, right this minute, to Be Your Becoming . . . now . . . go get yours.

MOVING CORE-WARD

YIPPEE! CONGRATULATIONS!!

It takes a lot of courage and heart to walk through the fire and come out on the other side, transformed. Buy yourself flowers today! Take yourself out on the town, or throw a Self-Centered Soirée for you and your friends. You've earned it.

Take a moment to reflect on how far you've come in a very short time. How do you feel you have shifted now, from where you were on Day 1? Many people never even take one step toward this spectacular way of being. You've just taken 21 gigantic leaps.

I hope I've helped you plant some seeds that you can grow into an even more dedicated healing lifestyle. Your Yoga Body, mind, and heart, will stick around as long as you stick with it.

I'm here for you beyond these three weeks for sure. Please consider me as your lifelong awesomeness advocate. There are many resources at the end of this book to help you keep studying with me, but I also suggest you find some local teachers/studios you like and surround yourself with a supportive in-person community that has your best interest in mind.

As you move core-ward, which is to say forward, from the calm strength of center, I invite you to stay in touch. I've created a sizzlingly fierce and inspiring Yoga Body community online, at www.21DayYogaBody.com. Stop by; you'll find a continual source of inspiration and dedication.

You'll meet some of the people in the book as we offer you many more Yoga Body recipes, lifestyle tips, and encouragement to keep you going during the book and beyond. You can find any of the products I suggest in the book on the site, too. It's one-stop shopping for your body and soul.

Last, but just as major, on our 21-Day Yoga Body blog you will be able to ask me all of your questions, share how you're using (or morphing) the book's offerings, and gain many more tools by getting to know new members of your Tribe—some even in your area.

I designed this online experience to be easy, and fun, for you to move not back to the way things were before you started the program but directly into a new lifestyle of mindfulness, passion, inner strength, and health. I can't wait to see how you transform as you go.

So until we meet again, keep on being the rock star you are, and always were . . . and keep building those empires, baby!

I'm with you all the way.

XO,
Sadie

RESOURCES

I'd love to stay in touch and continue your progress together!

I've got a ton of resources, free and otherwise, that you can use to get fit, navigate life, turbo-boost success, and look and feel fiercely fantastic. They will become a new support network for you, so you'll always keep moving forward, even after your 21-day program ends. Check out:

www.21DayYogaBody.com: Your VIP site for tons of book extras, videos of the yoga sequences, As to your Qs, my favorite yoga gear, food and drink suggestions, new recipe ideas, and so much more.

www.SadieNardini.com: My central hub for all things me, from new yoga workouts and online trainings to my calendar of events and a weekly blog you don't want to miss! Sign up for my newsletter here, too, so you won't miss a thing.

www.youtube.com/sadienardini: My online YouTube channel, where you'll gather tips and yoga vids, and watch me as I rock and roll all around the world bringing you the latest trends in fitness, wellness, food, and, of course, vino.

www.Facebook.com/SadieYoga: I post live updates, cool links, and awesome sauce on this page all day long—you can stop by to get a quick fix, have a laugh, or join the ongoing conversation. If you like it, be sure to "like" it!

www.Twitter.com: My Twitter handle is SadieNardini, all one word. Join me for short-form check-ins that no one else but my Tweeps get to see.

ACKNOWLEDGMENTS

If I thanked all the people separately who made this book possible, the list would be taller than the Empire State. That's because it's built entirely on the support and love of countless students, clients, and, really at this point, my extended family of birth and of choice, who, through their consistent attention, have made it possible for me to live my dreams.

So, if you're reading this . . . thank you, thank you, thank you. I could not have done any of this without you, nor would I want to. May this book help your lives become as magically delicious as you've helped to make mine.

More specifically, I offer insane amounts of gratitude to the following people. Please read through and take a moment to send some good vibes their way. They humbly gave of their time and energy to lift me up into the world so you could see me at all and benefit from this program: My mother and co-dreamer, Janet Parrish, a true visionary who taught me that it's not only possible but preferable to walk to the beat of a different drum, and who introduced me to the Universal ways at an early age. My agent, road wife, and best friend, Ava Taylor, who redirects my fires into manifestation and turns my crazy schemes into realities that are much better than I could have even imagined. My adventure partner and cover photographer, Tyler, for teaching me what it means to be in a conscious relationship, creating miracles out of dedication, and inspiring my heart beyond borders. This is some NLS!

Big huge thanks to Laurel Attanasio for her refinements on the final edit, JC Wang for a million hours of work so that I could shine, and

Curli Chan for jumping in at the eleventh hour to take so much off my plate and onto hers. Stephanie Tade, my literary agent and friend, a woman who truly walks the walk—and makes a mean chutney too. And, of course, to Sydny Miner, my editor, whose absolute understanding of and pure excitement about the project kept me going and whose laser clarity chipped away at the epic block of rock I handed her until it was sculpted into the sleek program you see before you. Thank you for navigating my process and for being there every step of the way! I've said it before and I'll say it again: you're a total rock star!

To the entire team at Random House, who spent their precious time and energy making sure you, dear reader, can find this book, and that it looks incredible. I'll never forget any of you. You're in my heart forever.

INDEX